Guray Demir
Aysegul Kusku
Gulay Eren

The effects of spinal anaesthesia on cerebral oxygen saturation

AF153183

Guray Demir
Aysegul Kusku
Gulay Eren

The effects of spinal anaesthesia on cerebral oxygen saturation

LAP LAMBERT Academic Publishing

Impressum / Imprint

Bibliografische Information der Deutschen Nationalbibliothek: Die Deutsche Nationalbibliothek verzeichnet diese Publikation in der Deutschen Nationalbibliografie; detaillierte bibliografische Daten sind im Internet über http://dnb.d-nb.de abrufbar.
Alle in diesem Buch genannten Marken und Produktnamen unterliegen warenzeichen-, marken- oder patentrechtlichem Schutz bzw. sind Warenzeichen oder eingetragene Warenzeichen der jeweiligen Inhaber. Die Wiedergabe von Marken, Produktnamen, Gebrauchsnamen, Handelsnamen, Warenbezeichnungen u.s.w. in diesem Werk berechtigt auch ohne besondere Kennzeichnung nicht zu der Annahme, dass solche Namen im Sinne der Warenzeichen- und Markenschutzgesetzgebung als frei zu betrachten wären und daher von jedermann benutzt werden dürften.

Bibliographic information published by the Deutsche Nationalbibliothek: The Deutsche Nationalbibliothek lists this publication in the Deutsche Nationalbibliografie; detailed bibliographic data are available in the Internet at http://dnb.d-nb.de.
Any brand names and product names mentioned in this book are subject to trademark, brand or patent protection and are trademarks or registered trademarks of their respective holders. The use of brand names, product names, common names, trade names, product descriptions etc. even without a particular marking in this works is in no way to be construed to mean that such names may be regarded as unrestricted in respect of trademark and brand protection legislation and could thus be used by anyone.

Coverbild / Cover image: www.ingimage.com

Verlag / Publisher:
LAP LAMBERT Academic Publishing
ist ein Imprint der / is a trademark of
OmniScriptum GmbH & Co. KG
Heinrich-Böcking-Str. 6-8, 66121 Saarbrücken, Deutschland / Germany
Email: info@lap-publishing.com

Herstellung: siehe letzte Seite /
Printed at: see last page
ISBN: 978-3-659-61611-2

MONITORING THE EFFECTS OF SPINAL ANESTHESIA ON CEREBRAL OXYGEN SATURATION IN ELDERLY PATIENTS WITH NEAR-INFRARED SPECTROSCOPY

Autor

Guray Demir M.D

Co-Autors

Aysegul Kusku, M.D
Gulay Eren, Assoc.Prof.,M.D.

Table of Contents

Abbreviations

Regional Cerebral Oxygen Saturation...rSO_2

Near Infrared Spectroscopy...NIRS

Cerebrospinal Fluid...CSF

Cerebral Blood Flow...CBF

Electromyografy...EMG

Cerebral Oxygen Diffusion...cDO_2

Cerebral Oxygen Content...CaO_2

Cerebral Metabolic Rate for Oxygen...$CMRO_2$

Partial Arterial Oxygen Pressure...PaO_2

Intracranial Pressure...ICP

Cerebral Perfusion Pressure...CPP

Transcranial Doppler...TCD

Jugular Venous Saturation...SjO_2

Arteriojugular Oxygen Gradient...$AjDO_2$

Cerebral Oxymeter...CO

In-vivo Optic Spectroscopy...INVOS

Systolic Blood Pressure...SBP

Diastolic Blood Pressure ....DBP

Mean Arterial Blood Pressure ....MAP

Heart Rate...HR

INTRODUCTION

Spinal anesthesia is a regional anesthesia method forming temporary block in spinal nerve roots by applying local anesthetic drugs into subarachnoid space and it has had an increasing popularity. Comparatively it may have superiorities over general anesthesia in some instances. It has a great number of advantages for prevention of protective reflexes such as continuation of spontaneous ventilation throughout the operation, patient's being awake, swallowing, coughing, continuation of postoperative analgesia and reduction in the duration of hospital stay (1,2). Spinal anesthesia has become a preferable method in many approaches since its effect commences fast and it is easily applicable. Of primary interferences, there are lower abdominal, inguinal, urogenital, rectal and lower extremity surgeries (3,5). In addition, it is used more securely in patients with allergic history to general anesthetics, malignant hyperthermia suspicion, muscle diseases and in patients with a full stomach requiring emergent interventions, and so forth (6).

The main aim of spinal anesthesia is to restore sensorial and motor blockade, however, the sympathetic denervation is regarded as a side effect generally causing systemic changes (3). Along with the advantages of spinal anesthesia, it has also some complications including hypotension, headache, nausea, vomiting, urinary retention, low back pain, neurological sequela, and meningitis. Hypotension depending on spinal anesthesia is the most frequently encountered complication. Systemic vascular resistance and cardiac output decrease based on sympathetic blockade and hypotension develops when bradycardia and reduction of contractibility are added. Hypotension particularly in elder patients can lead to a number of problems revealing cerebral ischemia developed by tissue hypoxia, myocardial infarction, acute renal deficiency and cardiac arrest (3,5).

Elder population has become the world's most rapidly increasing age group with enhanced life quality. People aged 65 and over are considered as old; 80 and over are regarded as elder population (7). Though spinal anesthesia application in old patients ensures some advantages during and after operation such as protection of cognitive functions, reduction of intraoperative bleeding, less postoperative thromboembolism and providing postoperative effective analgesia compared to general anesthesia, it can also introduce some disadvantages including bradycardia and late mobilization as well (8-14). While cardiac

4

output reduction and hypotension induced by spinal anesthesia effect does not impair hemodynamics to a large extent, these effects lead to a specific impact particularly on cerebral flow. Hypotension in old patients particularly aged over 60 with lower cardiac reserve indicates to decrease cerebral flow prominently (15), on the other hand, this issue is still contradictory in the studies published in the literature (16).

The virtual aim of neuromonitorization is both to protect neurological functions and supply optimal conditions giving opportunity to form a progress. Cerebral oximeter is a monitor used for the measurement of regional cerebral oxygen saturation (rSO2) and it functions with noninvasive near infrared spectroscopy (NIRS) technique. The monitor, not requiring flow or pulse for measurement, can show not only the balance between oxygen supply and need in brain tissue but can also indicate rSO2 in target ograns (17). In this study, it was aimed to search at what level the blood pressure alterations associated with spinal anesthesia to be applied in a standard protocol for elder patients affect cerebral blood flow and cerebral oxygenation.

GENERAL INFORMATION

A. SPINAL ANESTHESIA

History

Isolating alkaloid in the crystalized form by Albert Niemann in 1860 from coca leaf which has been chewed by South African natives for centuries for pleasure due to its sympathetic stimulant effects was the first important epitome of regional anesthesia. Twenty years later, attention of medical world turned to this agent with the publication of cocaine's all pharmacological effects. Heinrich Quincke mentioned spinal puncture for the first time in 1891 and developed Quincke needle referred by his name (18,20).

First central regional anesthesia applications were carried out by Bier and Tuffier in 1899 by using cocain. It was utilised in a wide variety of operations until the world war II, however, the use of regional anesthesia methods reduced owing to concerns regarding its neurological impairment possibility and since general anesthesia applications became more reliable due to the technological developments. In 1940, Walter Lemmon described continous spinal anesthesia with local anesthetic injection from a rubber tube with the help of a needle placed into the subarachnoid space (21). Tuohy designed lumbal needle for intradural catheterization during the same year. In 1944, Tuohy executed the first continuous catheterization attempt with 15G huber needle into the intrathecal space by pushing forward a number 4 urethral catheter (22).

Central regional anesthesia started to become popular after more effective and reliable local anesthetics were put into use in 1970s and the method was appreciated with better understanding (19).

Anatomy

Vertebral column consists of 33 vertebrae (Figure 1). These are divided into five regions; seven of them are cervical, twelve of them are thoracic, five of them are lombar, five are sacral and five coccygeal. Cervical vertebrae are the the narrowest part of spinal canal and their spinous processes are horizantal. Thoracic vertabrae form joints with the ribs. Their spinous processes are oblique and successive. Lombar vertebrae are the largest bone structures of the spinal column. Their spinal processes are nearly horizontal. Sacral vertebrae constitute fusion within the sacrum. There are nerve outflows out of the dorsal and ventral foramens. Coccyx comprises fusion of the 3 or 4 rudimentary vertebrae. The line connecting both iliac cristae usually passes from the spinous process of L4-5. Spinous processes of vertebrae are used as reference points in determining the level in anesthesia applications (23).

Ligaments found in the vertebral column line up from front to back as ligamentum longitudinale anterior, ligamentum longitudinale posterior, ligamentum flavum, ligamentum interspinosum and ligamentum supraspinale. Ligamentum flavum is a strong link composing of yellowish elastic fibers which combine vertebral arcus. It is right above the duramater. The space between ligamentum flavum and duramater is the epidural space, and it is called as the subdural space between the dura and the arachnoid membrane. Epidural space ends with the foramen magnum. Spinal subdural space is associated with the cranial subdural space. Therefore, resistance by ligamentum flavum during the intervention and loss of resistance are important in terms of understanding the localization of the needle (18, 19, 24).

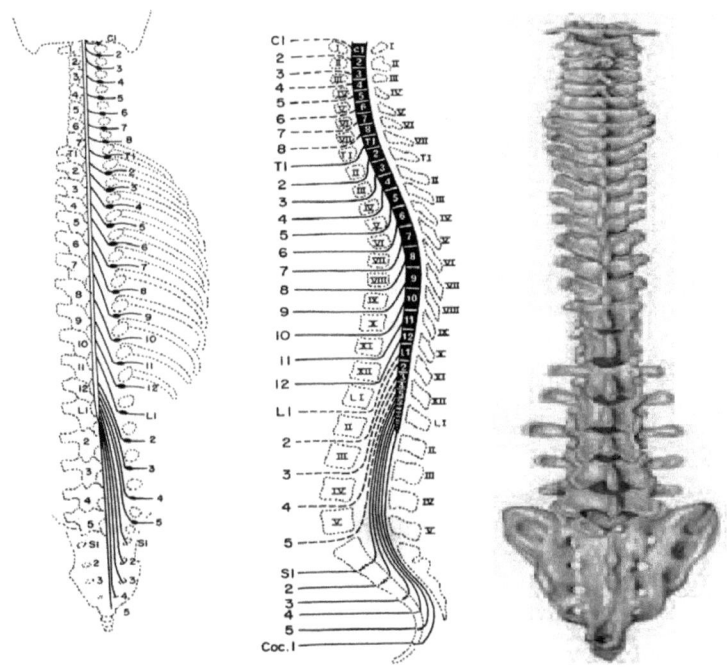

Figure 1. Vertebral Column Anatomy

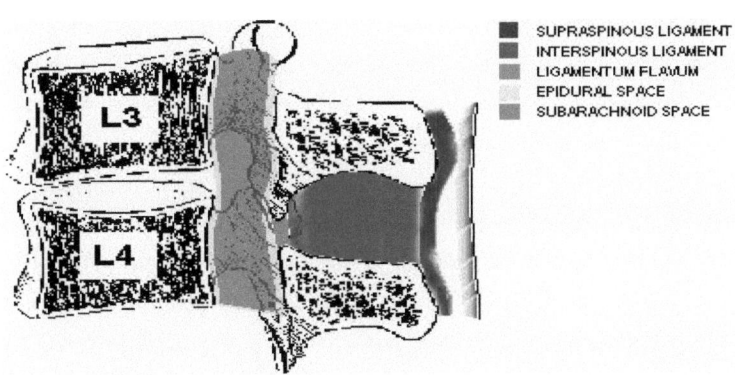

SUPRASPINOUS LIGAMENT
INTERSPINOUS LIGAMENT
LIGAMENTUM FLAVUM
EPIDURAL SPACE
SUBARACHNOID SPACE

Figure 2: Vertebral column ligaments

Spinal Cord

Spinal cord lies within the spinal canal. Dura mater, fatty tissue, venous plexus and the meninx surround the cord. There are epidural space, veins and fatty connective tissue in the most outer region of the brain. Dura, the most external membrane of the spinal cord, is a leakproof intensive tissue and it protects the spinal cord (Figure 3). Dura mater is associated with the intracranial dura. Spinal cord ends at L1-2 level in adults. It can sometimes end at L1 or L2 vertebral body level, rarely at T12 and even at L3 level. In children, however, it ends at the level of lower border of L3 vertebra at birth; it ends at the lower border level of L2 body and it reaches at the level of L1 body until 12-16 years of age, that is, the level of adults'. The roots of anterior and posterior spinal nerves unite in the intravertebral space. They leave the intervertebral foramen as spinal nerve (19, 24, 25). Spinal cord is 40-45 cm long, 1 cm wide and it is flat from anterior to posterior. It continues with medulla oblongata on the top. It ends as conus medullaris at the level of L2. The extension beginning from the edge of conus medullaris proceeding to the bottom of os coccygis is called as filum terminale.

Spinal meninges are located from exterior to interior as dura mater, arachnoid and pia mater. The distance between outer surface of dura mater and bone is called as epidural space. The distance between interior surface of dura mater and exterior surface of arachnoid's inner lamina is called as subdural space. The distance between the interior surface of inner lamina of arachnoid and exterior surface of piamater is called as subarachnoid space. Pia mater having an extensive network of vessels sticks firmly to the exterior surface of medulla spinalis and covers all indentations and pedicles. Arachnoid, on the other hand, jumps from one pedicle to another; it never lines indentations (19, 24, 25).

Meninges have two separate parts; one of them is in the cavum cranium and the other one is in canalis vertebralis. Dura mater, medulla spinalis and dura mater spinalis wrapping its radixes fastens on foramen magnum and it continues with dura mater encephali. The lower part, however, begins from conus medullaris, proceeds all the way down to the filum terminale by wrapping it and ends by getting the name of infundibulum dura at 2nd sacral vertebral level. The extensions emerging from inner surface of pia mater enter into medulla spinalis. Subarachnoid distance involves spinal nerve roots, denticulate ligament, spongiform reticulum of fibrils connecting arachnoid to pia (19, 20, 24).

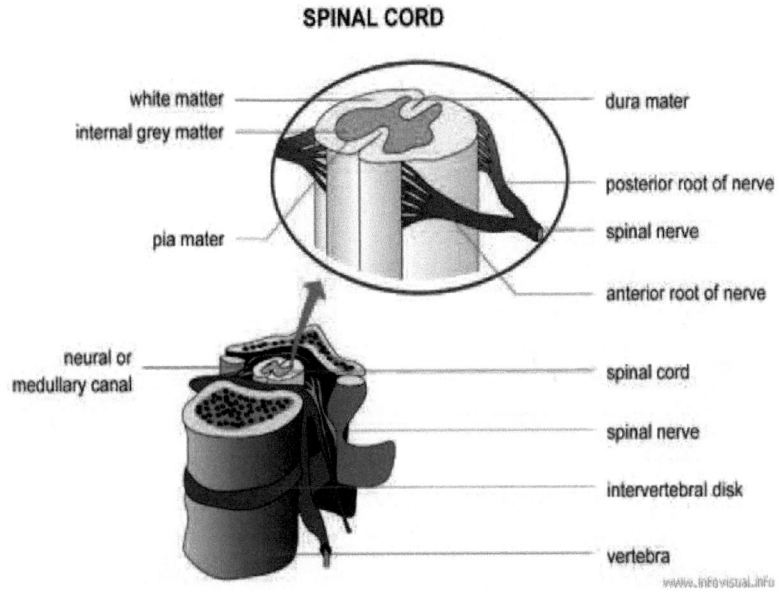

Figure 3: Spinal Cord

Cerebrospinal Fluid (CSF)

Cerebrospinal fluid is found in the spinal and cranial subarachnoid spaces and brain ventricles. CSF is as much as 100-150 cc. CSF forms by secretion or ultrafiltrations of choroid plexus located in lateral-third and fourth ventricles. It is resorbed by meninx vein plexuses and lymphatic veins (19, 24).

CSF content :

Intensity: 1.006 (1.003-1.009)

Volume: 120-150 ml (in spinal space 25-35 ml)

Sodium: 133-145 mEq/lt

Potassium: 2,5-3 mEq/lt

Chloride: 118-132 mEq/lt

Phosphorus: 1,6 mg/dl

Magnesium: 2 -2,5 mEq/lt

Calcium: 2-3 mEq/lt

pCO2: 48 mmHg

HCO3: 23mmHg

Protein: 23-38 mg/dl

Pressure 60-80 mmHg

pH: 7.32 (7.27- 7.37)

Blood Supply of Spinal Cord

Arterial System:

Posterior spinal artery derived from cerebral arterial system has prosperous collaterals and feeds posterior grey and white substance of the spinal cord. Its collaterals are subclavian, intercostal, lumbal and sacral arteries. Owing to these prosperous collateral anastomoses, in segmental arterial injuries no cord ischemia is seen in areas which this artery feeds. Anterior spinal artery forms by attaining a branch of every vertebral artery and it is the only artery progressing in the midline falling amongst the medulla oblangata pyramids. It extends downwards in the anterior longitudinal sulcus of spinal cord. It provides numerous branches into and around the spinal cord. The biggest one among them is radicularis magna or Adamkiewicz artery. It often enters into medulla spinalis at the level of L1 in the left side between T8 – L3. It feeds lumbar segments and lower thoracic area (19, 20, 24).

Venous system :

It extends through all medulla spinalis both in vertebral channel and outside of it. Plexus located around the medulla spinalis flows into venosus vertebralis internus and externus and from there, it also pours into vv. vertebrales, vv. intercostales, vv. lumbales, vv. sacrales lateralis (24).

Nervous innervation of the meninges: The posterior part of dura and arachnoid does not involve nerve fibrils. Therefore, no pain is felt when dura is perforated. The anterior part is innervated by the sinovertebral nerves (19, 24).

The Physiology of Spinal Anaesthesia

The aim of the central blockage is to prevent pain and loosen the skeleton muscle. According to the duration of surgery, local anesthetic agent is chosen. The physiological reaction to central blockage is determined with somatic and visceral afferent and efferent innervation. Local anesthetic agent, mixing the cerebrospinal fluid, affects the spinal nerve roots. The distribution of local anesthetic agent in CSF depends on the gravity of the substance, CSF pressure, patient's position and solution's heat (25).

When local anesthetic agents are mixed with the cerebrospinal fluid, its diffusion reduces and its movement to central nervous system slows down gradually. For neural blockage, the penetration of the local anesthetic agent into the lipid membrane is required and it must block the sodium channels in the axoplasm. Following subarachnoid injection, local anesthetic agents affect nerve trunks which are 2 cm above the intervertebral foramens. Since motor fibers are affected by the local anesthetic agent more difficultly and slowly, sensory block resides longer compared to motor block and it generally ascends two segments higher than the motor block (25).

Nerve fibers are of three types (A, B, C). A type nerve fibers have subgroups such as α (alpha), ß (beta), γ (gamma) and δ (delta) (Table 1).

Table 1

Type	Effect	Myelin	Nerve Size	Cm
A α	Motor	+	++++	++++
A β	Soft touch, Pressure	+	+++	+++
A δ	Pain, Heat, Touch	+	+++	++
A γ	Muscle tone	+	++	+
B	Preganglionic sympathetic fibers	+	++	+
C	Pain, Pressure	-	+	+++

11

Somatic structure is a part of sensory system; overall sensorial information from body surface and deep structures is transferred by somatic sense. This information is carried to medulla spinalis, bulbus, pons, reticular matter of mesencephalon, thalamus and sensorial areas of cortex.

Type A and B nerve fibers are typical fibers of spinal nerves with myelin. Type B fibers have smaller diameter and separate from type A fibers by displaying negative back potential following their stimulation. Type B nerve fibers are preganglionic autonomous nerve fibers (26).

Since type C nerve fibers have no myelin and they are very thin, they transfer impulses at low speed. Most peripheric nerves are composed of type C nerve fibers that form more than half of the sensory fibers. Type C nerves account for postganglionic autonomic fibers, as well. They carry sensory information of body surface. All sensory messages from somatic segments of body enter into medulla spinalis from dorsal roots. Entering into the medulla spinalis, a large part of thick sensory nerve fibers (A beta fibers) pass immediately to posterior cord and go up throughout the medulla spinalis. Sub-branches coming from thinner sensory fibers (C and delta A fibers) and thicker fibers form synapses with posterior horn cells. Ventral and lateral spinothalamic pathways commence from this point. These pathways account for spinothalamic system. Spinothalamic system is constructed by thick nerve fibers with too much myelin and transferred to the brain with a speed of 35-70 m / sec (26).

Spinal posterior cord system: (26)

1. Touch sensations requiring the localization of stimulus to a large extent
2. Touch sensations requiring light severity grading
3. Phasic sensations such as vibration sensations
4. Sensations informing the movement which affects them on the skin
5. Kinesthetic sensations
6. Pressure sensations regarding the evaluation of fine distinctions of pressure intensity

Spinothalamic system: (26)

1. Pain
2. Hot and cold sensations

3. Insensible touch and pressure sensations that can slightly localize and differentiate severity differences on body surface

4. Itching and tickling sensations

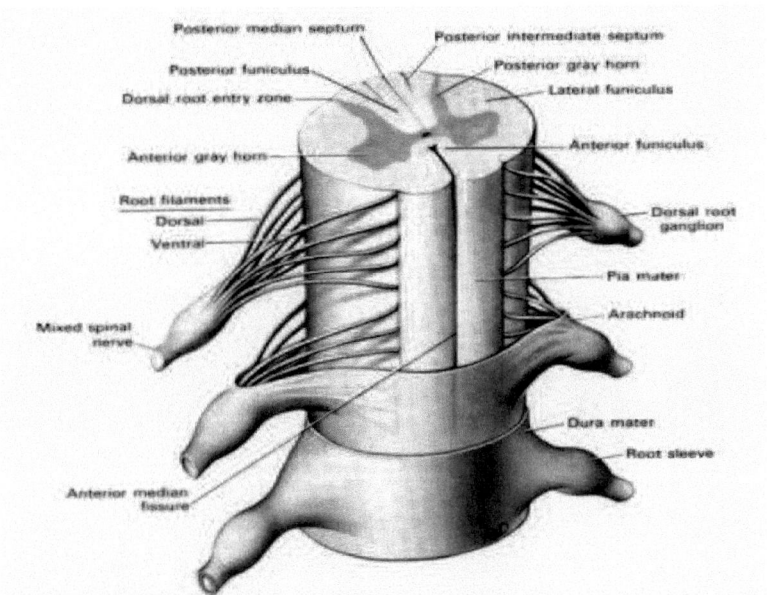

Figure 4: Spinal structure

Segmenter Sensation Areas: Dermatomes

Every spinal nerve innervates a segmenter area called as dermatoma in the skin. There are no definite boundaries among adjacent dermatomes. In a posterior root damage corresponding to whole segment of spinal cord, there can be a destruction with a profound loss in sensation. Nerves leaving vertebral colon show a particular spread and make up dermatomes. Dermatomes should be known in order to determine anesthesia level in spinal anesthesia and evaluate the complications. In a spinal cord divided by segments by spinal couples, there are 31 spinal nerves in total, involving eight cervical, twelve thoracic, five lumbar, five sacral and one coccygeal (20, 25).

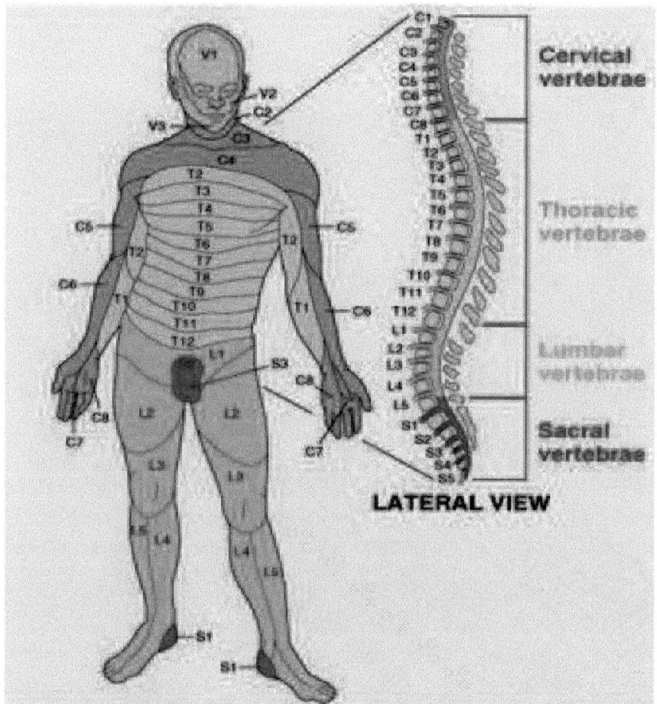

Figure 5: Dermatomes

Spinal reflexes are also used in determining the anesthesia level of a patient: Epigastric (T 7-8), abdominal (T 9-12), cremasteric (L 1-2), knee (L 2-4), plantar (S 1-2), ankle (S 1-2). These spinal reflexes guide us in the evaluation of dermatomes affected by local anesthetic agents (27). Bromage scale is used in establishing the motor block level.

Bromage scale:

0: No paralysis, patient can literally bring his/her foot and knee to flexion.

1: Patient can only move his/her knee and feet but cannot lift them firmly.

2: Patient cannot bend his/her knee but can only move his/her feet.

3: Total paralysis.

14

The transmission of pain to central nervous system

Pain signals are transmitted by thin delta type A (3-20 m/sec.) and B (0.5 -2 m/sec.) fibers. By compressing nerve body to a reasonable extent without blocking C fibers, delta type A fibers are blocked. With this blockage, pain resembling pinprick vanishes. C type thin nerve fibers transmit burning and grip type pain. After a fast pinprick type pain, a burning pain occurs one second later. Pinprick pain informs about the agent giving damage to the person and thus it is effective in drawing the person away from the stimulus that causes pain. Gradually developing burning pain sense tends to create much more pain and leads to an excruciating pain suffering. If C fibers are blocked without blocking delta fibers with low dose local anesthetic agents, pain resembling grip disappears. Pain sense belonging to visceral organs is transmitted by C type sensorial fibers of sympathetic nerves in chest and abdomen cavities (25).

SPINAL ANESTHESIA

Spinal anesthesia is one of the frequently used and oldest regional anesthesia techniques. The injection of local anesthetic agent into subarachnoid space causes a temporary block in nerve transmission in nerve roots and paralysis in autonomic, sensational and motor fibers. The application of spinal anesthesia is easy and its effect initiates fast. The quality of anesthesia is excellent. There is no systemic toxicity. The area that surgical intervention will be carried out, intervention duration and type, necessary muscle relaxation degree, illnesses accompanying and estimated blood loss are the factors determining the choice of spinal anesthesia application (28).

Spinal anesthesia can be used in all surgical interventions under the umbilicus level. As a result of splanchnic sympathetic blockage at T5-L1 level, parasympathetic tone domination and correspondingly contraction in small intestines and relaxation in sphincters occur. This impact provides good surgical conditions with the relaxation of abdominal wall (19). It has advantages such as perfect muscle relaxation and postoperative analgesia quality, increase in intestinal motility, thromboembolism prophylaxis due to sympathetic blockage, suitability to outpatient interventions and easy monitorization. Nevertheless, spinal anesthesia is ineligible in upper abdominal surgeries. Since there is no vagus and phrenic nerve blockage, it has disadvantages including nausea, vomiting and hiccup.

Spinal Anesthesia Indications

- Lower extremity surgeries
- Perineal surgeries
- Lower abdominal surgeries
- Urologic endoscopical surgery
- Rectal surgery
- Obstetric surgery
- Vascular surgery (19, 20, 23, 25).

Spinal Anesthesia Contraindications

- Patients with whom cooperation cannot be made and who fear too much, patients with mental disorders and psychological issues.
- Cardiovascular System Diseases: Hypovolemia (due to hemorrhage, sepsis, shock), severe anemia, coronary artery diseases, coronary sclerosis, cardiac decompensation. Aortic and other valvular diseases are considered as relative contraindications.
- Systemic infections such as generalized sepsis and bacteremia, AIDS and local infections in areas where spinal anesthesia is applied.
- Nervous System Diseases: Brain tumours, meningitis and other central nervous system infections. Spinal cord and peripherial nervous diseases, poliomyelitis, multiple sclerosis, demyelinating illnesses.
- Patients receiving anticoagulant treatment; relatively heparin, aspirin and other antiplatelet drug use.
- Congenital anomalies of spinal cord, scoliosis, metastatic tumours of vertebral colon after laminectomy.
- Specific intraabdominal conditions such as increased abdominal pressure, extensive upper abdominal surgical intervention, prolonged surgery (relative) and intestinal obstruction.
- Resistance that surgeon shows to conscious patient are involved in relative contraindications (19,20,23,25).

Patient's position

- Sitting position: It is the most frequently utilised and the easiest position. However, its use is restricted in hip fractures, pregnant women and patients that cooperation cannot be established.
- Lateral decubitis: It is used in hip and leg fractures. Optimal flexion of spine is ensured by holding patient's shoulders and hip.
- Prone position: It can be preferred in surgeries such as rectum, sacrum and lower part of the vertebral colon. Due to gravity, CSF does not drip but can be aspirated (19, 25).

Process

- Approach from midline: Interlaminar foramen is surrounded by a bonuos circle and covered with ligamentum flavum. If the direction of needle is inappropriate, it can reach at any place of this circle bone. While the direction of the needle must be vertical in lower lumbar spaces, it must be slightly inclined to cephal in upper spaces.
- Paramedian approach: It is preferred in situations when lomber puncture cannot be performed from midline. Vertebral colon does not need too much flexion. Shoulders and arms are straightly held. The needle tip is pushed forward as it will be extending from midline at 1-1,5 cm length to lateral caudal by providing 80°angle with skin and its tip will be 4 cm deep from the skin. The most common error performed in this technique is to direct the needle extremely to cephal (28).
- Taylor technique: It is a paramedian injection with lumbosacral approach performed at L5 level which is the widest space. After the patient is brought to flexion in lateral decubitis or sitting position, it is entered with 12 cm spinal needle from 1 cm medial and 1 cm caudal to the lower point of spina from posterior superior iliac crest. The needle is pushed forward with 55° angle medially and cephally (19, 20).

Spinal Anesthesia Types

- **Low spinal anesthesia:** It involves lower thoracic, lumbar, sacral segments. Level does not ascend over T10. Hip is also anesthetized. It is carried out from L2-3 level.
- **Saddle block:** It is the blockage of lower lumbar and sacral segments. L3-S3 dermatomes are affected. This block is formed when local anesthetic agent is given in the sitting position from L 4-5 space, and following this process, the patient should be kept waiting in sitting position at least for five minutes.
- **High spinal anesthesia:** It is performed from the level of T4-12. The block over T4 is considered to be the highest spinal block. Hypotension is apparent. There is a respiratory insufficiency possibility.
- **Unilateral spinal anesthesia (hemiblock):** This type of block is applied to patient by giving lateral decubitus position according to local anesthetic agent's osmolarity. The block occurs after keeping the patient in the same position at least for 5 minutes.
- **Total spinal block:** This type of block is not an anesthetic block type. It is a complication formed after the block going up too high in spinal anesthesia performed. The depression of bulbar centers is the point in question. Consisting a block in the cranial nerves such as in peripheric nerves occur with the deterioration of circulation as a result of autonomic imbalance between sympathetic and parasympathetic systems (29, 30).

The Preparation of Patient:

The preparation of the patient begins with briefing in anesthesia. Patients must be informed about their spinal anesthesia and its results. The process must be initiated after patient's consent is obtained. Disapproval of process by the patient is involved in the contraindications of spinal anesthesia. Overall physical examination of the patient must be made including cardiovascular system, respiratory system and neurological system. Vertebral colon must be evaluated. Infections, scars, anatomic disorders should be noted. Lumbar interspinous spaces should be palpated. Total blood count and coagulation parameters of the patient must be controlled. Severe anemia aggravates the effects of hypotension occuring after spinal anesthesia. Coagulation parameters are important in terms of probable complications in coagulopathic situations. Fear of patients should be eliminated prior to operation during the preanesthetic visit. If necessary, sedation can be performed with oral or intramuscular benzodiazepines.

Safety:

All equipment must be prepared for spinal anesthesia as if general anesthesia would be performed; entire monitorization must be carried out. The use of electrocardiography, blood pressure and SpO$_2$ monitoring ensures early awareness in case of collapse (19, 20).

COMPLICATIONS

Cardiovascular complications:

Preganglionic sympathetic fibers come out of T1-L2 segments. The cardiovascular effect of a block below L2 is minimal. When block reaches to T1-L2, complete sympathetic denervation develops. It is influenced by cardiovascular fibers leaving from T1-T4. The most important effects of sympathetic block are on cardiovascular system. Arteries and arteriolles are dilated, systemic vascular resistance and arterial pressure decrease. Tonus loss occurs in veins and venules, as well.

As veins cannot protect their tones, they dilate on a large scale. Venous capacity increase and blood accumulation in veins decrease venous return. Reduction in venous return leads to a significant drop in cardiac output and blood pressure. The safety of spinal anesthesia is only provided by the protection of venous return. Cristalloid treatment is important in hypotension treatment. Prior to a spinal anesthesia to be performed from medium and high level, applying 500-750 cc of cristalloid solutions rapidly is beneficial.

Bradycardia: It develops by the blockage of preganglionic cardioaccelerator (T1- T4) fibers and distention receptors in the right heart. Bradycardia is also dependent on the decrease of pressure of large veins entering into the right atrium (19, 20).

Decrease in coronary blood supply: In conjunction with reduction in mean arterial pressure, coronary pressure also decreases. Oxygen requirement of myocardium increases prominently (19, 20).

Cerebral circulation: It is widely known that normal aging process leads to cardiovascular system changes. In addition to advancing age, it has been proven that cerebral blood supply (CBS) decreases owing to changes formed by age in cerebral vessels. Besides, the cerebral autoregulation impairment also contributes to CBS decline. According to results released in literature, the effect of spinal anesthesia on cerebral oxygenation is contradictory and studies related to this issue have accelerated with the development of neuromonitorization. Cerebral blood supply is kept at normal limits as long as mean arterial pressure drops below 55-60 mmHg (19, 20).

Renal circulation: Renal blood supply is affected less by decline in the blood pressure (5).

Hepatic circulation: Spinal anesthesia has no distinct effect on hepatic blood supply, oxygenation and drug metabolism until T4 level is reached (19,20).

Respiratory complications :

A spinal anesthesia ascending until thoracal dermatomes can lead to paralysis in the intercostal muscles. Diaphragm compansates for paralysis in intercostal muscles. However, this compensation is impossible in patients with lung disease and high intraabdominal pressure, obeses, pregnants, in extreme upside-down positions.

Patients gone through high spinal anesthesia cannot cough owing to the paralysis of their abdominal and chest wall muscles. Their closing volumes have reduced. Atelectasia can develop. If motor block reaches to C 3-5 level, apnea can arise since phrenic nerve is influenced by the paralysis. Respiratory arrest develops mostly due to sedative drugs, obesity, ventilation/perfusion inconsistency, hypotension in the respiratory center and ischemia because of decline in cardiac output. Therefore, fixing cardiac output will enable respiratory problems to be corrected. During high spinal anesthesia, a distinct change does not happen in their arterial blood gases. No significant change occurs in tidal volume, maximal inspiratory volume, negative intrapleural pressure. Nevertheless, a prominent decrease occurs in maximum respiratory capacity and maximum expiratory volumes. In the course of expiration, impairments form in the respiratory mechanics (19, 20).

Headache:

Headache can develop whenever a lumbar puncture is performed. The thickness of the needle, gender (the incidence is more likely to be seen in women), age (more common in young) and early mobilization are risk factors. It is an increasing pain by standing up and frequently prevalent in frontal or occipital areas. It develops in most patients within 3 days following spinal anesthesia. It is considered that brain is deprived of its cushion as a result of CSF leakage and headache develops by enabling susceptible structures to be strained. Headache can be taken under control by using a small scale needle (>22G), minimizing the diameter of hole through being paralel with dura fibers of needle's tip, hydration and bed rest in postoperative period. In addition; use of analgesics, abdominal bandage, prevention of constipation and epidural blood patch are also beneficial (19, 20).

Neurological Complications :

A severe and permanent impairment in spinal anesthesia is uncommon. Neurological impairment can be caused by ischmea, direct trauma or the chemical effects of local anesthetic. The primary cause of spinal cord ischemia is hypotension. The prevention of probable hypotension protects spinal cord from ischemia.

Watching over sterile conditions, avoiding spinal anesthesia in patients with systemic disease possessing neurological symptoms, choosing hot sterilization instead of neurotoxic substances in the sterilization of ampuls and abstaining from drugs with high toxicity and density decrease this probability. Epidural hematoma likely to be due to any cause can lead to neurological complications. Traumatizing a nerve root during an injection results in a neurological damage (19). Persistant paresthesia and motor weakness are the most frequently seen neurological complications. Paraplegia and impairment of cauda equina roots are rare.

Chronic adhesive arachnoiditis and cauda equina syndrome are the most important neuroloical complications. Cauda equina syndrome occurs with the diffuse injury of lumbosacral nerve roots. It can arise with one dose injection of dibucaine, procaine, mepivacaine and tetracaine into subarachnoid space (31). Local anesthetic spread is limited with the use of microcatheter use in continuous spinal anesthesia, sacral- perianal anesthesia prolongs and cauda equna syndrome can occur. Administring lidocaine continuously through spinal catheter and with high doses into subarachnoid space can lead to cauda equina syndrome (32). Nevertheless, block is restricted with catheter malposition and drug maldistribution (33). Cauda equina syndrome or other neurological injuries are not solely dependent on catheter (26). Of the potential reasons of cauda equina syndrome, there are direct and indirect traumas, ischemia, infection and neurotoxic reactions (31, 35). Cauda equina syndrome can de identified with specific symptoms such as saddle block, bowel-bladder sphincter dysfunction and paraplegia (34).

Medical history should be obtained at full detail to differentiate whether neurological disabilities are the complications of regional anesthesia or not. If a patient is suspected to have neuropathy, s/he should be taken into consideration and preoperative evaluation should be carried out with neurological examination. Electromyography (EMG) can be helpful in this issue.

Others

Vomiting – Nausea : Cerebral hypoxia occurs depending on organ contraction during hypotension or surgical opeation. Vomiting-nausea complaint can be prevented by delivering oxygen to patient and fixing hypotension or treated. In sympathetic blockage on T6 segment, nausea and vomiting are seen more frequently (19).

Urinary retention : In regional anesthesia, bladder function is removed with the blockage of S 2-4 segments. Bladder dysfunction occurs with the blockage of efferent parasympathetic fibers innerving m. detrusor vesica and the inhibition of bladder drainage. The function returns by unblocking (19).

Back and waist pain : They can be based on puncture and also result from relaxation of back muscles and unsupported waist (19). There can be postoperative back pain due to contraction of interlumbal and joint capsules of lumbosacral ligaments, recovery of lumbal convexity, relaxation of paraspinous muscles. Back pain can particulary develop with lithotomy position.

Infection : Infection incidence is reduced by paying attention to antisepsis/asepsis rules in use of materials.

Hypothermia : Peripheric vasodilatation developed by sympathetic blockage, affecting heat regulation by local anesthetics that pass into circulation, peripheric heat detection impairment developed by the inhibition of afferent thermoreceptor fibers found in spinal cord, thermosensitive affection in spinal cord with the application of cold local anesthetic agents lead to hypothermia (36).

B. CEREBRAL PHYSIOLOGY and ITS METABOLİSM

Energy metabolism in brain has several unique pathways and they are dependent on oxygen and glucose. Therefore, they are based on continuous blood flow to fulfill these needs. Oxygen gets into circulation via simple difusion through alveolar-capillary membrane in alveoles. This incident is dependent on partial pressure difference of oxygen. Oxygen is carried into blood in two ways : independently and as dependent on hemoglobin. Partial oxygen pressure in capillary are higher than PaO_2 in tissues. As a result of this, oxygen carried in plasma separately from hemoglobin is obtained by simple difusion. In consequence of oxygen lost from plasma, PaO_2 decreases and O_2 dependent upon hemoglobin breaks free (37, 38, 39).

Cerebral oxygen amount (CaO_2) and cerebral blood flow (CBF) are determiners of cerebral oxygen distribution (CDO_2). As it occurs in tissue hypoxemia, reduction takes place in CDO_2 due to hypoxemia on highest degree or hemoglobin decline. While the utilization speed of brain tissue ($CMRO_2$) reduces in coma, it increases with convulsion, hyperthermia and neurotransmitters coming out related to first impairment. Compared to other tissues, brain tissue is more vulnerable to ischemia since its relaxation energy need is higher and it has no oxygen store (40, 41, 42). Normal CBF is 30–70 mL/100g/min. Impairment in neuronal function begins to form when CBF drops under 20 mL/100 g/min (43).

The major determiners of brain's blood flow are arterial blood pressure (PaO_2), arterial carbondioxide pressure, pressure autoregulation and neuronal stimulation's degree.

23

CBF increases in hypoxia and hypercapnia. Unless PaO2 lowers under 50 mmHg, CBF is not influenced. Nevertheless, even a 1 mmHg change in carbondioxide leads to 3-4% change in CBF. The effect of carbondioxide in question is fairly significant. Because hypercapnia in a patient with brain edema can cause herniation or intracranial pressure (ICP) can diminish with hypocapnia. Cerebral autoregulation is the protection of CBF based on blood pressure changes. When average blood pressure (ABP) is between 50-150 mmHg, CBF can be kept fixed. If average blood pressure drops further, CBF reduces. The best identifier of CBF is cerebral perfusion pressure (CPP). CPP is equal to the difference of ABP and cerebral venous pressure. When ICP increases, the difference between ABP and ICP can be calculated since cerebral venous pressure is determined with ICP. To provide sufficient CBF, it will be appropriate to keep CPP at approximately 70 mmHg and ICP below 20 mmHg (44,45).

The difference between CMRO2 arterial oxygen content and jugular venous oxygen content can be calculated. Oxygen saturation measured with the help of oxymetrical catheter to be placed into jugular vein allows cerebral venous content and thereby CMRO2 to be estimated. While CMRO2 increases with neuronal activity, convulsion and fever, it decreases with hypothermia, barbiturates and benzodiazepines (47,48,49).

C. NEUROMONITORIZATION

The actual purpose of neuromonitorization is to protect neurological functions and provide optimal conditions that will enable a chance to form an improvement. While the bedside measurement of CBF was inappropriate until 1948, CBF was started to be calculated after Kety and Smith had discovered CT method developed by xenon. Nonetheless, this method only provides momentary CBF and does not ensure continuous monitorization. Transcranial doppler (TCD) is used by neurologists to evaluate bedside cerabral blood flow today and this method evaluates CBF indirectly. 2 methods are utilised for direct continuous measurement. They are laser doppler flowmetry and thermal diffusion (50).

Arterial oxygen allows cerebral oxygenation. Thus, cerebral oxygenation monitorization has been the target of neurologists for many years. The principal methods used accordingly are jugular venous saturation follow-up and transcranial cerebral oximetry (51).

Transcranial Doppler (TCD) :

Although TCD as a non-invasive method based on a measurement technique depending upon ultrasonic principals of cerebral blood flow is attractive, some technical difficulties in its practice inhibit its common use. Of these difficulties, they are prob localization and keeping it fixed in the same place during entire operation. The most appropriate bone window is usually ensured by at the level of temporal bone mastoid process and medium cerebral artery blood flow can be measured with this angle (52-54).

Jugular venous saturation follow-up :

Jugular venous saturation (SjO2) is a parameter reflecting the balance between cerebral oxygen delivery and consumption. Cerebral oxygen consumption CMRO2 is described as cerebral metabolic rate for oxygen and it is calculated by the difference between cerebral blood flow (CBF) and arteriojugular oxygen odds (AjDO2) : CMRO2 = CBF x AjDO2. If arterial oxygen saturation, hemoglobin concentration and CMRO2 are stable, SjO2 is directly proportional with cerebral blood flow and it gives an idea about global cerebral oxygenation. SjO2 = CBF/CMRO2. AjDO2 is normally found in a narrow space such as 4-9 ml/dl and being less than 4 ml (SjO2>%75) means that it is above the requirement and being further than 9 ml (SjO2<%54) means that the flow cannot meet the need. Thus, global ischemia diagnosis is possible with the continuous SjO2 monitorization. It has become possible to follow the case with an optical reader catheter placed in the area concerned instead of spaced sampling from the tip of catheter put in jugular bulbus. These kind of catheters are placed as retrograde from jugular internal vein and the tip of catheter must be placed right beneath the middle ear floor in order to prevent the contamination of blood coming from extracranial formations. Pushing forward the tip of catheter 15 cm is adequate (54-56).

Transcranial cerebral oximeter

The imaging techniques of central nervous system have reached advanced technology today. However, these imaging techniques have improved about neurological anatomy and structural impairments. The demanded level associated with the functions of central nervous system has not been reached yet. The potential use of cerebral oximeter (CO) for the monitorization of cerebral oxygenation and near-infrared spectroscopy (NIRS) were first   suggested   by   Jobsis   in   1977.

Cerebral oximeter used in the sectional oxygen saturation is a monitor functioning with NIRS technique. It does not require pulse or flow. It shows the oxygenation and perfusion of target organ by reflecting capillary sample (57). Cerebral oximeter that has been used since the middle of 1970's is a technique monitorizing the balance between the cerebral oxygen delivery and its consumption in noninvasive and constant way (58). In vivo optical spectroscopy (INVOS) device used in this technology is based on the principle that every material is a characteristic light absorbance. Hemoglobin, cytochrome c oxidase known as cytochrome aa3 enzyme, are main chromophores in NIRS (materials absorbing light in specific frequencies) (57). Near infrared spectroscopy measures the proportion of oxyhemoglobin to total hemoglobin in a region below the sensor based on the relative permeability difference of a biological tissue to near infrared light. This ratio is described as a percent value of rSO2 (59, 60). NIRS, reflecting the cerebral tissue oxygenation, monetarizes intraparenchymal in frontal cortex and oxygenation in microcirculation (61). Cerebral oxymeter is a reliable indicator of cerebral oxygenation changes caused by hypoxemia (62). The index values of hypoxemia, hypocapnia, hypercapnia and arterial hypotension reflect cerebral oxygenation (63). This is method has been used owing to different reasons such as carotid endarterectomy causing hypoxia, dislocation of endotracheal tube to the right main bronch or to determine arterial obstruction (64, 65). In many processes including perioperative monitorization, peripheral perfusion can be useful by evaluating non-invasively. Some researchers have shown that cerebral oximeter can be used in ischemic extremity monitorization as well (66).

Harel et al (67) determined forearm tissue saturation change rate through reactive hyperemia with NIRS by measuring tissue saturation changes after ischemic period and comparing strain gauge plethysmography with radionuclide plethysmography. Ono et al (68) reported that cerebral oxymetry functions compatible with single photon emission tomography in determining vasospasm in 5 patients gone through subarachnoid hemorrhage and INVOS monitorization can be superior than other monitorization systems in displaying oxygen in vasospasm region.

Two sticky pads placed on forehead involve both light source and receiver. Electrodes radiate through near infrared wave length between 730 nm and 810 nm. They measure

26

oxygenized / deoxygenized hemoglobin rate at 730 nm wave length and sosbestic point (oxygenized / deoxygenized hemoglobin transition point) rate at 810 nm wave length. They measure total tissue by oxygenation offering total light transmission index, arithmetic difference in the reflecting signal severity. Normal values are at 58-82% in healthy people. Different spaces of two receiver sensors are important points and they are placed in 3-4 cm lateral of light source. Since there is a relationship between tissue penetration depth and reflecting light incidence, they provide the measurement of cortical oxygenation by differentiating extracerebral tissue signal from intracerebral tissue signal and sensors' gap difference (69). Oxygenized / deoxygenized hemoglobin rate is measured and regional hemoglobin saturation in frontal cortex is attained by subtracting surface signal from deep signal (70). As a result of algorithmic analysis used, it can be stated that a balance is ensured between cerebral oxygen delivery and and its consumption in normoxic, hypoxic, hypocapnic conditions without a major change (71).

The signals from two hemispheres are transmitted to screen thanks to sensors placed on forehead. Only data from deep part of brain are shown by subtracting signal from proximal receptor from distal receptor. The big number on the screen displays continuing basal brain oxymeter values and small number, however, displays basal brain oxymeter values. Beam spreading from sensory analyses blood in the form of micro vessel (for example; arterioles, venules, and capillary) with help of venous/arteriel blood volume which is approximately ranging from 70 to 30 %. Therefore, cerebral tissue oxygen saturation values are generally lower than arterial oxygen saturation values or pulse oxymeter SpO2 values and higher than brain venous oxygen saturation (for example; cephal catheter, internal jugular oxygen saturation values) (72).

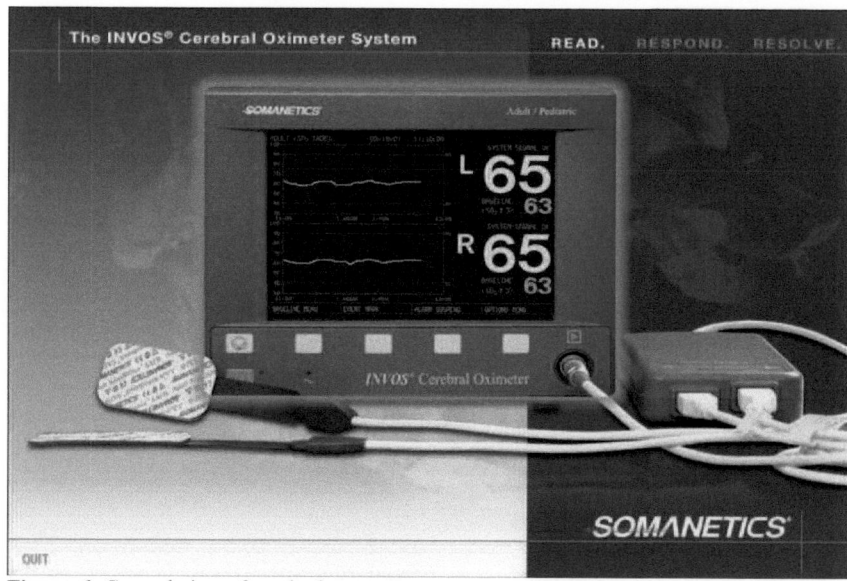

Figure 6: General view of cerebral oxymeter

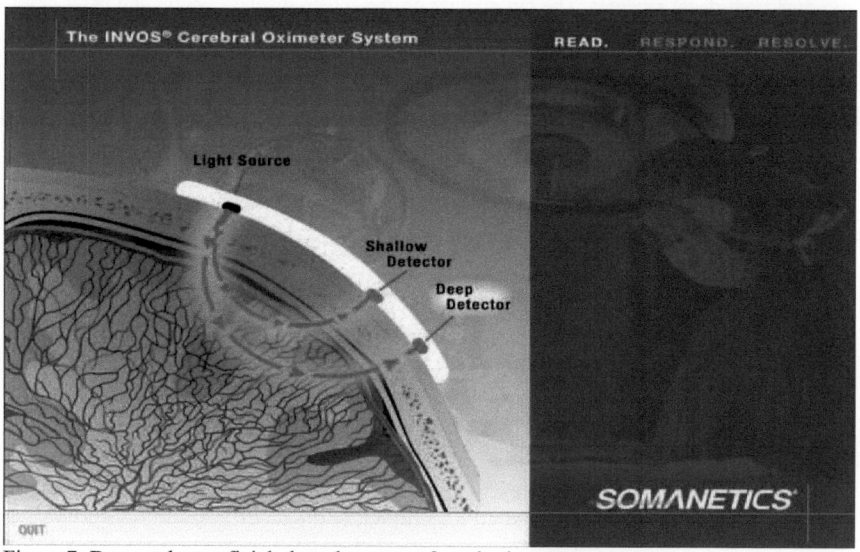

Figure 7: Deep and superficial photodetectors of cerebral oxymeter sensory

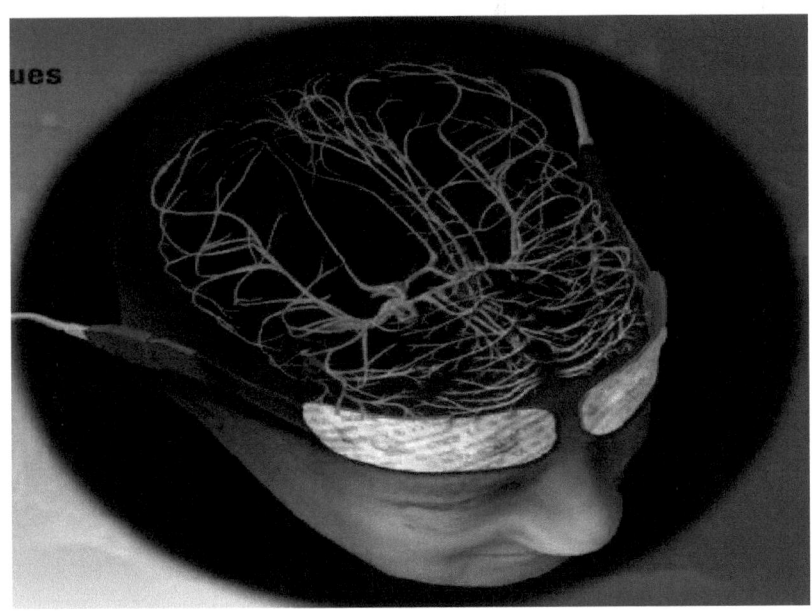

Figure 8: Placing cerebral oxymeter sensory on forehead

MATERIAL and METHOD

Our study was applied in a total of 25 cases aged 60 and over in American Society of Anesthesiologists (ASA) I-II risk groups who were planned to have urology, cardiovascular andgeneral surgery operation and preferred to have spinal anesthesia by obtaining research ethics committee approval from Bakırköy Dr. Sadi Konuk Training Research Hospital Anesthesiology and Reanimation Department. All patients involved in the study were signed informed consent form. Individuals with mental and neurological disease, congestive heart failure, anemia, hematologic disorders, bleeding that can affect htc level, bleeding inclination (prothrombin activity lower than 67.5%, bleeding duration > 3 minutes, prothrombin time > 13 seconds, thrombocyte count< 100000), electrolyte imbalance and liquid deficit were not involved in the study. The patients who had been applied spinal anesthesia, however, their sensorial block level was insufficient with "pin-prick" test and therefore had been applied general anesthesia were excluded from the study.

The patients were visited in the evening before the operation and informed about the procedure to applied to them. The cases that had potential conditions to form contraindication for regional anesthesia practice and did not accept it were not involved in the study. When patients were taken into preoperative preparation room, they were monitorized and basal values of systolic blood pressure (SBP), diastolic blood pressure (DBP), average blood pressure (ABP) and cardiac apex beat (CAB), peripherical oxygen saturation (SpO2), cerebral oxygen saturation (with Somanetics İnvos Oximeter 5100C :Somanetics Comp. 1653 East Maple Road, Troy, MI, USA trademark and model device) were recorded. Patients were taken into operation room after their venous pathways had been opened with 18-20 G peripheric vein cannula. SBP, DBP, ABP, CAB, rSO2, SpO2, SS values were recorded. After the skin had been cleaned by following antisepsis rules in sitting position and covered, intratecal blockage was carried out by entering into subarachnoid space from L3-L4 interspace with 22-25 no "Quincke" needle by standard technique and equal amount local anesthetic (15 mg buvicain 3 ml). Patients were positioned as lying back following the spinal anesthesia . Sensorila block levels of cases were recorded according to dermatomes with "pin-prick" method in thr first 10 minutes (3-5-10. minute).

No medication that could affect cognitive findings in preoperative period were applied. Standardized mini-mental test (SMMT) was applied to patients by the same physician to evaluate cognitive functions in an hour time before and after the operation. Scores that had been obtained were recorded. After spinal anesthesia had been applied, surgical intervention was permitted following 30 minute adequate sensory block (at surgical onset VAS<20 mm) or if necessary motor block had been waited to be formed. Following the puncture, hemodynamic parameters were followed at each minutes during preoperative 60 minutes. In this period and in the course of surgical intervention, patient's blood pressures, cardiac apex beats, peripheral oxygen saturations, respiratory rate, cerebral oxygen saturation (by somenetics invos cerebral oximeter method) were evaluated and recorded by noninvasive oscillometric method. According to values measured basally in blood pressure, the patient was planned to be treated with 3 minutes intervals if it decreased lower than 30% or lower than 90 mm Hg systolic pressure and if diastolic pressure reduced lower than 40 mmHg, 5 mg ephedrine was decided to be applied until diastolic pressure reached at normal values. Treatment was intended to be applied with 3 minute intervals until cardiac apex beat reached 50 beat/min value by 0.5 mg atropine in case cardiac apex beat dropped below 40 beat/min. The data obtained were evaluated statistically. The changes in blood pressure and correlation of cerebral oxygenation changes was analysed.

Statistical Research

While the data obtained from study were evaluated, NCSS (Number Cruncher Statistical System) 2007&PASS 2008 Statistical Software (Utah, USA) programme was used for statistical analyses. As a result of power analysis when difference was accepted as 12 and deviation was 10 in an assessment performed by the Sol rSO2 measurement average, sample number was determined as 23 in groups whose values were established as power : 0.90, β:0.10 and α:0.01.

Measurement periods were taken as a mutual variant (covariant) to determine the connection between rSO2 and ABP measurements and generalized linear regression analysis was applied. When evaluating study data, Spearman's Rho Correlation Coefficient was used for the relationship analysis among parameters for the comparison of quantitative data as well as descriptive statistical methods (Average, Standard deviation). Significance was assessed at the level of $p<0.05$.

RESULTS

The study was carried out with 25 patients; 76% was male (n=19) and 24% was female (n=6). The ages of cases ranged from 60 to 77 and the average was 62,80±4,38 years.

Table 2: ABP Measurements

MAB	Min-Max	Avg±SS
Basal	85-144	114,88±16,10
5 minutes	79-132	106,64±13,38
10 minutes	78-128	100,16±14,23
15 minutes	74-126	97,32±14,61
20 minutes	73-119	92,52±13,66
25 minutes	70-120	89,88±13,38
30 minutes	70-119	88,60±13,20
40 minutes	69-116	86,40±12,90
50 minutes	68-107	84,88±11,13
60 minutes	68-107	83,80±11,71
F		97,62
p		0,0001

ABP measurements were as indicated in Table 2.

Significant changes were observed statistically (p=0,0001) amid ABP measurements which were obtained as basal and at 5, 10, 15, 20, 25, 30, 40, 50, 60 minutes intervals. Periods creating significance were reported in Nevman Keuls multiple comparison test.

ABP value graphic being in tendency to drop continuously according to basal value was shown in Figure 9.

rSO$_2$	Sum of squares	Degree of freedom	Mean square	F	P
ABP	240,429	1	240,429	7,740	0,006
Measuremen Times	2853,631	9	317,070	10,207	0,001
Residual	15190,591	489	31,065		

	rSO$_2$/ ABP
R^2	0,291
Corrected R^2	0,269

To determine the relationship between rSO2 and ABP, measurement times were accepted as mutual variable (covariant) and generalized linear regression analysis was applied. Statistically significant relationship was observed in measurement times and between rSO2 and ABP (p=0,006, p=0,001). Corrected R2 value which identifies the level of relationship was found as 0,269.

Table 3: CAB Measurements

CAB	Min-Max	Avg±SS
Basal	55-111	78,20±11,32
5 minutes	57-108	75,92±11,06
10 minutes	60-107	74,80±10,69
15 minutes	57-100	73,92±10,22
20 minutes	59-96	74,04±9,57
25 minutes	57-93	72,56±9,82
30 minutes	56-92	72,08±9,15
40 minutes	56-90	72,20±9,35
50 minutes	57-91	72,40±9,21
60 minutes	57-90	72,04±8,76
F		9,79
p		**0,0001**

The distribution of CAB values of patients according to their measurement times were given in Table 3. Statistically significant change was observed (p=0,0001) in CAB averages at basal 5. minute, 10.minute, 15.minute, 20.minute, 25.minute, 30.minute, 40.minute, 50.minute, and 60. minute. Periods developed significance was indicated in Newman Keuls multiple comparison test.

Figure 10: CAB Measurements

rSO_2	Sum of squares	Degree of freedom	Mean square	F	P
CAB	225,330	1	225,330	7,246	0,007
Measurement Times	5023,388	9	558,154	17,950	0,001
Residual	15205,690	489	31,095		

	$RSO_2/$ CAB
R^2	0,287
Corrected R^2	0,268

Statistically significant relationship was observed in measurement periods and between sSO2 and CAB values (p=0,007, p=0,001). Corrected R^2 value signifying the level of connection was found as 0,268.

Table 4: SPO₂ Measurements

SPO_2	Min-Max	Avg±SS
Basal	96-100	98,53±1,04
5 minutes	95-100	98,52±1,15
10 minutes	97-100	98,36±0,99
15 minutes	96-100	98,24±1,05
20 minutes	96-100	98,36±1,18
25 minutes	96-100	98,52±0,96
30 minutes	96-100	98,32±1,03
40 minutes	96-100	98,44±1,04
50 minutes	96-100	98,40±1,08
60 minutes	96-100	98,32±0,94
F		0,82
p		0,598

SPO$_2$ measurements were as shown in Table 4. No statistically significant change was observed in SPO2 averages as basal at 5 minutes, 10 minutes, 15 minutes, 20 minutes, 25 minutes, 30 minutes, 40 minutes, 50 minutes, 60 minutes intervals (p=0,598). Periods identifying significance were established in Newman Keuls multiple comparison test.

rSO$_2$	Sum of squares	Degree of freedom	Mean square	F	P
SPO$_2$	26,235	1	26,235	0,854	0,356
Measurement Times	5310,238	9	590,026	19,207	0,001
Residual	15021,425	489	30,719		

	RSO$_2$/ SPO$_2$
R^2	0,285
Corrected R^2	0,251

No statistically significant relationship was observed between rSOs and SPO2 values (p=0,356), however, there was a statistically significant relationship in measurement periods (p=0,001). Corrected R2 value signifying the level of connection was determined as 0,251.

Table 5: Respiratory rate measurements

RESPIRATORY RATE	Min-Max	Avg±SS
Basal	9-16	11,40±1,58
5 minutes	10-16	11,44±1,44
10 minutes	10-18	11,56±1,66
15 minutes	9-17	11,24±1,56
20 minutes	9-16	11,40±1,35
25 minutes	10-17	11,68±1,57
30 minutes	10-17	11,60±1,70
40 minutes	9-17	11,32±1,67
50 minutes	10-18	11,36±1,63
60 minutes	10-18	11,52±1,58
F		1,31
p		0,230

Respiratory rate measurements were as shown in Table 5. There was no statistically significant change in basal respiratory rate averages at 5, 10, 15, 20, 25, 30, 40, 50, 60 minutes intervals (p=0,230). Periods producing significance in Newman Keuls multiple comparison test.

RSO$_2$	Sum of squares	Degree of freedom	Mean square	F	P
Respiratory rate	4016,188	1	4016,188	178,028	0,001
Ölçüm Zamanları	5549,788	9	616,643	27,334	0,001
Residual	11031,472	489	22,559		

	RSO$_2$/ SS
R^2	0,464
Corrected R^2	0,450

Statistically significant connection was observed in measurement periods and between rSO2 and respiratory rate values (p=0,001). Corrected R2 value determining the degree of connection was discovered as 0,450.

Table 6: Right rSO$_2$ Measurements

Right rSO$_2$	Min-Max	Avg±SS
Basal	54-78	65,04±6,75
5 minutes	55-74	64,08±6,23
10 minutes	52-74	62,84±6,28
15 minutes	52-73	61,64±6,08
20 minutes	51-71	60,56±5,81
25 minutes	50-69	58,88±5,41
30 minutes	50-68	57,68±5,03
40 minutes	49-68	56,96±5,00
50 minutes	48-67	56,32±4,96
60 minutes	46-67	55,76±5,01
F		127,8
p		**0,0001**

Right rSO2 measurements were as shown in Table 6. Statistically significant change was observed among Right rSO2 averages as basal at 5 minutes, 10 minutes, 15 minutes, 20 minutes, 25 minutes, 30 minutes, 40 minutes, 50 minutes, 60 minutes intervals (p=0,0001). Periods creating significance was reported in Newman Keuls multiple comparison test.

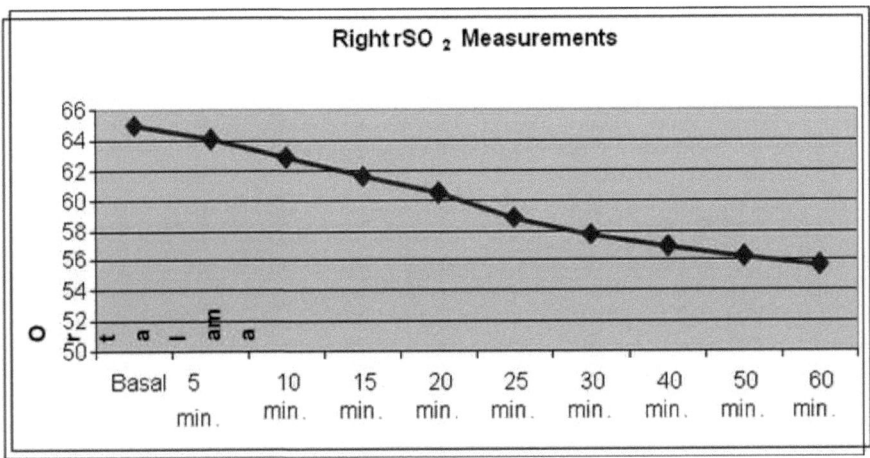

Figure: Right rSO₂ Measurements

According to basal values measured prior to spinal rSO₂ displayed a continuous decrease.

Table 7: Left rSO2 Measurements

Left rSO₂	Min-Max	Avg±SS
Basal	50-78	64,96±5,74
5 minutes	49-75	63,84±5,85
10 minutes	49-75	62,44±5,73
15 minutes	48-73	61,36±5,68
20 minutes	47-73	59,80±5,42
25 minutes	46-70	57,84±5,34
30 minutes	44-70	56,88±5,34
40 minutes	43-69	56,40±5,08
50 minutes	40-69	55,64±5,30
60 minutes	40-68	54,88±5,24

F	162,9
p	0,0001

Left rSO2 measurements were as shown in Table 7. Statistically significant change was observed amid Left rSO2 averages as basal at 5. minute, 10. minute, 15. minute, 20. minute, 25. minute, 30. minute, 40. minute, 50. minute, 60. minute intervals (p=0,0001). Periods creating significance were indicated in Newman Keuls multiple comparison test.

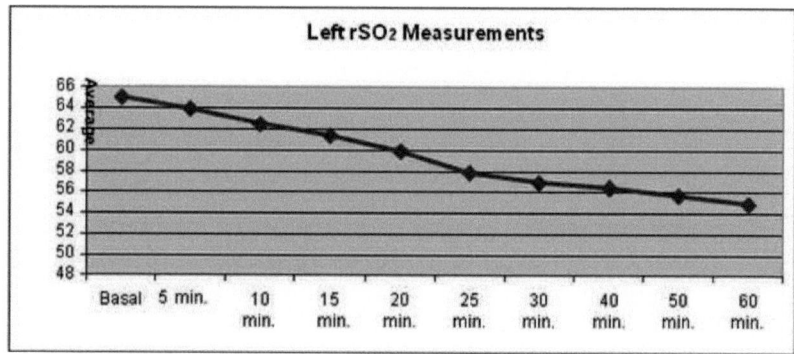

Figure: Left rSO₂ Measurements

Table 8: Right and Left rSO2 Comparison

Right rSO₂	Right rSO₂	Left rSO₂	t	p
Basal	65,04±6,75	64,96±5,74	0,086	0,932
5 minutes	64,08±6,23	63,84±5,85	0,27	0,789
10 minutes	62,84±6,28	62,44±5,73	0,44	0,664
15 minutes	61,64±6,08	61,36±5,68	0,339	0,737
20 minutes	60,56±5,81	59,80±5,42	0,818	0,422
25 minutes	58,88±5,41	57,84±5,34	1,266	0,218
30 minutes	57,68±5,03	56,88±5,34	0,968	0,343
40 minutes	56,96±5,00	56,40±5,08	0,797	0,433
50 minutes	56,32±4,96	55,64±5,30	0,929	0,362
60 minutes	55,76±5,01	54,88±5,24	1,31	0,203

No statistically significant difference was observed among rSO2 averages as basal 5minutes, 10 minutes, 15 minutes, 20 minutes, 25 minutes, 30 minutes, 40 minutes, 50 minutes, 60 minutes intervals (p>0,05).

Table 9: SMMT Scores

	Min-Max	Avg±SS
SMMT SCORE 1	15-27	18,44±2,53
SMMT SCORE 2	14-27	18,48±2,55
t		-0,44
p		0,664

The distribution of SMMT scores were as in Table 9. Statistically no significant change was observed between SMMT1 and SMMT2 scores (p=0,664).

Table 10: Relationship between Left rSO$_2$(%) Change Level and SMMT(%) Changes

Right rSO$_2$	SMMT (%) Change
5 minutes	0,031
10 minutes	0,009
15 minutes	0,149
20 minutes	0,190
25 minutes	-0,078
30 minutes	-0,061
40 minutes	0,031
50 minutes	0,169
60 minutes	0,077

r: Spearman's rho correlation coefficient

There was no statistically significant relationship between change levels seen in left rSO2 follow-ups and SMMT change levels (p>0,05)

Table 11: Relationship between right rSO₂(%) change level and SMMT (%) changes

Right RSO$_2$	SMMT (%) Change
5 minutes	-0,082
10 minutes	0,131
15 minutes	**0,430***
20 minutes	0,295
25 minutes	-0,050
30 minutes	-0,017
40 minutes	-0,147
50 minutes	-0,137
60 minutes	-0,171

r: Spearman's rho correlation coefficient

There was no statistically significant relationship between the change levels seen in right rSO2 follow-ups and SMMT change levels (p>0,05).

Newman Keuls Multiple Comparison Test	MAB	CAP	Right RSO2	Left RSO2
Basal / 5 Minutes	0,0001	0,001	0,001	0,0001
Basal / 10 Minutes	0,0001	0,001	0,0001	0,0001
Basal / 15 Minutes	0,0001	0,0001	0,0001	0,0001
Basal / 20 Minutes	0,0001	0,0001	0,0001	0,0001
Basal / 25 Minutes	0,0001	0,0001	0,0001	0,0001
Basal / 30 Minutes	0,0001	0,0001	0,0001	0,0001
Basal / 40 Minutes	0,0001	0,0001	0,0001	0,0001
Basal / 50 Minutes	0,0001	0,0001	0,0001	0,0001
Basal / 60 Minutes	0,0001	0,001	0,0001	0,0001
5 Minutes / 10 Minutes	0,001	0,076	0,001	0,001
5 Minutes / 15 Minutes	0,0001	0,004	0,0001	0,0001
5 Minutes / 20 Minutes	0,0001	0,026	0,0001	0,0001
5 Minutes / 25 Minutes	0,0001	0,002	0,0001	0,0001
5 Minutes / 30 Minutes	0,0001	0,002	0,0001	0,0001
5 Minutes / 40 Minutes	0,0001	0,001	0,0001	0,0001
5 Minutes / 50 Minutes	0,0001	0,005	0,0001	0,0001
5 Minutes / 60 Minutes	0,0001	0,007	0,0001	0,0001
10 Minutes / 15 Minutes	0,0001	0,067	0,0001	0,001
10 Minutes / 20 Minutes	0,0001	0,33	0,0001	0,0001
10 Minutes / 25 Minutes	0,0001	0,035	0,0001	0,0001
10 Minutes / 30 Minutes	0,0001	0,015	0,0001	0,0001
10 Minutes / 40 Minutes	0,0001	0,017	0,0001	0,0001

10 Minutes / 50 Minutes	0,0001	0,046	0,0001	0,0001
10 Minutes / 60 Minutes	0,0001	0,041	0,0001	0,0001
15 Minutes / 20 Minutes	0,0001	0,851	0,0001	0,002
15 Minutes / 25 Minutes	0,0001	0,149	0,0001	0,0001
15 Minutes / 30 Minutes	0,0001	0,043	0,0001	0,0001
15 Minutes / 40 Minutes	0,0001	0,055	0,0001	0,0001
15 Minutes / 50 Minutes	0,0001	0,126	0,0001	0,0001
15 Minutes / 60 Minutes	0,0001	0,087	0,0001	0,0001
20 Minutes / 25 Minutes	0,001	0,025	0,0001	0,0001
20 Minutes / 30 Minutes	0,0001	0,007	0,0001	0,0001
20 Minutes / 40 Minutes	0,0001	0,012	0,0001	0,0001
20 Minutes / 50 Minutes	0,0001	0,044	0,0001	0,0001
20 Minutes / 60 Minutes	0,0001	0,035	0,0001	0,0001
25 Minutes / 30 Minutes	0,01	0,524	0,0001	0,0001
25 Minutes / 40 Minutes	0,0001	0,614	0,0001	0,0001
25 Minutes / 50 Minutes	0,0001	0,829	0,0001	0,0001
25 Minutes / 60 Minutes	0,0001	0,568	0,0001	0,0001
30 Minutes / 40 Minutes	0,0001	0,78	0,0001	0,025
30 Minutes / 50 Minutes	0,0001	0,533	0,0001	0,0001
30 Minutes / 60 Minutes	0,0001	0,953	0,0001	0,0001
40 Minutes / 50 Minutes	0,019	0,533	0,0001	0,0001
40 Minutes / 60 Minutes	0,001	0,753	0,0001	0,0001
50 Minutes / 60 Minutes	0,035	0,308	0,001	0,0001

DISCUSSION AND CONCLUSION

Hypotension developed in patients who have been performed spinal anesthesia is the most commonly incountered complication of spinal anesthesia with 33% rate. Hypotension is dependent on systemic vascular resistance loss due to sympathetic block. Owing to dilatation formed in venules, venous capacity leads blood to accumulate in veins and thus causes reduction in cardiac output (3-5).

Cereabral blood flow and cerebral oxygenation are affected by Htc level, ABP, pO2, pCO2, CAP and SPO2 (44, 45). These parameters were followed in patient group over 60 year-old who had been applied spinal anesthesia in this study as well.

Some studies carried out in animals and humans indicated that as a result of drop in blood oxygen level, CBF increases to provide sufficient oxygen to brain. Reduction in oxygen delivery to cerebral tissue can be dependent upon drop in oxygen level amount or decrease in

41

Htc level. Acceptable Htc level is reported as 21% for brain perfusion in old population (77-79). There was no patient that had adequate bleeding to affect Htc level in our study group.

Sympathetic blockage developed during spinal anesthesia leads to hypotension. Numerous researcher has performed many studies on the complication ıf spinal anesthesia since the beginning of its first application. In a study in which tetracaine and bupivacaini were compared by Edström and Blitt in 1986 (87), it was reported that an apparent hypotension was observed in both groups, however, reduction in ABF was more significant in tetracaine group. In a study in which bupivacain and mepivacain were compared by Bengtssan and Edström (86) in 1983, it was shown that a significant hypotension was observed in both groups, but there was more decrease in mepivacain group. The effects of developed hypotension on hemodynamic were started to be shown more clearly. In a study carried out by Mc Crae AF, Wildsmith (88) in 1993, it was determined that thanks to transthoracic echocardiogram, systemic vascular resistance, cardiac index and cardiac apex beat decreased in patients who had been applied spinal anesthesia. In a study in which low dose bupivacain and high dose bupivacain were compared by Karim Asehnoure and Eric Lorousse (89) in 2005, it was informed that although cardiac output was found higher in patients who had been performed spinal with low dose bupivacain, an obvious decrease was displayed in cardiac output. In a study in which lateral decubitus and supin position were compared in a spinal anesthesia by Kelly and Mc Coyd (90) in 2005, it was shown that lateral decubitus position prolongs hypotension formation period and it also decreases total vasoconstructor myrrh used. Development of imaging methods with technology enabled effects of hypotension and accompanying hemodynamic changes on organ systems to be observed more explicitly . In a study in which cerebral oxygenation had been analyzed in geriatric group patients to be performed hip operation by David Hoppestein and Edna Zohar (91) in 2005, they observed that rSO2 decreased according to basal value and defended that it developed due to reducing cardiac output. In a study carried out by Vincent Minville and Karim Asehnounne (92) in 2009, however, they investigated the impacts of spinal anesthesia in old patients on cerebral blood flow. In their study where people over 60 were compared with those under 60 year-old, they used TCD method and they determined that CBF was lower in people over 60. It was maintained as a cause that degeneration occurs in cerebral vessels with advancing age and impaired autoregulation could not compansate for hypotension developed during spinal anesthesia. In a study fulfilled by Nishikawa and R. Hagiwara'nın (93) in 2006, however, as a result of sedation score composed in patients after administeration of spinal block by using two different dose bupivacain, they compared cerebral oxygenation by utilising BİS and via cerebral oximetre. While the first group was composed of patients with high spinal block (T6 and over) who had been apllied 2,7 ml 0,5% bupivacain, the second group was composed of those with block level lower than T12 and who had been applied 1,5 ml 0,5% bupivacain. As a result, they determined that regional cerebral oxygen supply reduced in patients who had been applied spinal anesthesia in the first minute. This change was undetected in the patient group who had been applied low level block. In our study, however, of the ABP averages statistically significant change was observed in patients who had been applied spinal as basal at 5 minute, 10 minute, 15 minute, 20 minute, 25 minute, 30 minute, 40 minute, 50 minute, 60 minute intervals (p=0,0001). We can attribute the correlation between cerebral oxygenation and ABP to degeneration developed in cerebral vessels and impaired autoregulation developed as a result of uncompensated hypotensive attack and eventually reduction of CBF.

The number of CAB affects cerebral blood flow and cerebral oxygenation. In a study carried out by İde K. and Boushel in 2000, they showed that bradycardia which was developed in patients whom had been applied beta-1 blocker and unilateral stellate ganglion blockage reduced MCA blood flow via transcranial doppler method (73). In a study carried out by İde K and Pott F in 1998, they indicated that MCA blood flow rate by using TCD and NIRS method is dependent upon cardiac output (80). In another study conducted again by İde K and Gullon AL (1999), they showed that cardiac output decreased as a result of atrial fibrilation developed during exercise and thus MCA blood flow rate reduced (81). Bradycardia developed during spinal anesthesia occurs related to blockage of preganglionic accelerator cardiac fibers. The higher the level of dermatoma in which block develops, this risk increases (3-5). It was observed in our study that the count of minute CAB reduced in all patients who had been followed by our team, however, bradycardia which was at the lifethreatening level or required treatment. Statistically significant change (p=0,0001) in patient group that we followed was observed among CAB averages as basal at 5. minute, 10. minute, 15. minute, 20. minute, 25. minute, 30. minute, 40. minute, 60. minute. Statistically significant relationship was observed between rSO2 and CAB values and in measurement times (p=0,007, p=0,001). Corrected R2 value specifying the level of relationship was found as 0,268. We can attribute the data obtained to decreasing cardiac output owing to arising bradycardia.

Respiratory functions are not affected in spinal anesthesia on a large scale in blocks at T7-10 dermatoma level. Respiratory minute count, end-tidal CO_2, PaO_2, $PaCO_2$ values do not change. Respiratory functions and diaphragmatic compensation whose innervation is with N. Frenicus are not affected in blocks up to T4. Patients in high spinal anesthesia cannot cough owing to paralysis of chest wall and abdominal muscles. Therefore, they can develop atelectasia (75-76). Cerebral blood flow is affected by PaO_2 and $PaCO_2$. Reduction of blood oxygen concentration leads to increase of CBF. Todd MM, Wu B, Maktabi M (82) showed in their studies that cerebral blood flow rate increases in hypoxia and hemodilution condition. In a study conducted by Hino A and Ueda S. (83), they demonstrated that CBF increased by using TCD method in patients whose blood hemoglobin level reduced and therefore cerebral oxygen delivery decreased. Statistically no significant change (p=0,598) was observed in patients that spinal had been applied among SPO2 averages as basal at 5 minutes, 10 minutes, 15 minutes, 20 minutes, 25 minutes, 30 minutes, 40 minutes, 50 minutes, 60 minutes intervals. Block level developed in patients is not effective on their respiratory functions. There was no statistically significant relationship (p=0,356) between rSO2 and SPO2 values but statistically significant relationship was seen in measurement periods (p=0,001). Corrected R2 value signifying the level of relationship was found as 0,251. We thought that this meaningful correlation between SPO2 and rSO2 was caused by reduction in rSO2 in its measurement periods.

Cognitive dysfunction can be described as loss of memory and intellectual skills. Of the factors increasing cognitive dysfunction risk after surgery, the most common ones are hypotension and hypotermia. Standardized mini-mental test is a screening test evaluating cognitive functions as quantitative and it was reported that it is preferred in studies since it is valid, reliable, short and it can be applied before and after the surgery and it is easy to perform (96). SMMT is a test used in the determination of cognitive function impairment, diagnosis pahse and follow-up of treatment. Total score is 30. The score of every problem is written in the application form of the test. High scores show that activation is less and there is a better cognitive function (97). In a multicenter study conducted by Gustavson Y and Berggren D (94) in 1998, they indicated that hypoxia and hypotension are the biggest risk factor in cognitive dysfunction developed after major surgery in old patients. In a study carried out in old patients in 1990, it was shown that cognitive dysfunction observation risk was higher compared to general anesthesia following regional anesthesia in patients to be applied arthroplasty (95). It was reported that this impairment in cognitive functions was dependent on the degree of hypotension and its duration. In our study, however, no significant difference

44

was found between SMMT before and after spinal and evaluated cognitive function scores (p>0,05).

In conclusion; hemodynamic changes developed during low level intrathecal anesthetic agent application in old patients negatively affect cerebral oxygenation. It has become possible to determine impaired cerebral oxygenation balance thanks to advancing new imaging methods even though hemodynamical changes developed in the course of spinal anesthesia do not provide symptoms clinically.

SUMMARY

Objective: Hypotension particularly formed due to spinal anesthesia in elder population can lead to a range of problems such as cerebral ischemia, myocardial infarction, acute renal insufficiency developed by tissue hypoxia. The effects of hypotension occured in older patients who had been applied spinal anesthesia were aimed to be determined on oxygenation with cerebral oximeter.

Methods: A total of 25 cases 60 and over 60 year-old American Society of Anesthesiologists (ASA) I-II risk group whose lower extremity and abdominal surgery had been planned with spinal anesthesia were included in our study. Basal cerebral oxygen levels were determined with cerebral oxymeter method followed by standard monitorization application. SMMT was performed by the same physician for two times, prior to and after the operation, to determine the cognitive function level of patients. Intrathecal blockage was performed with standard technique and equal amount local anesthetic (5,15% mg bupivacain). Sensorial block level of cases was recorded to dermatomas with "pin-prick" method in first 10 minutes (3-5-10. minute). Hemodynamic parameters following puncture and cerebral oxygen levels were recorded every 5 minutes during peroperative 60 minutes.

Results : Statistically significant change was observed between ABP and CAB averages of patients. The relations of values with rSO2 were connection with rSO2 was established. determined with Newman Keuls multiple comparison test. No significant change in other parameters followed and significant

45

Conclusion : When data obtained from the study were evaluated, it was determined that hemodynamical changes formed before and after the application affected oxygenation in a negative way even if low dose intrathecal aneasthetical agent was used in old group patients.

REFERENCES

1. Albright G, Forster R. Spinal analgesia-physiolgic effects. In: Collins VJ (Ed.). Principles of anesthesiology. 3rd ed. Philedelphia: Lea & Febiger; 1993. p.1445-570.

2. Atkinson RS. Spinal analgesia. In: Atkinson RS, Rushmman GB, Davies NJH (Eds.). Lee's synopsis of anaesthesia. 11th ed. Oxford: Buttenvort-Heinemann International Edition; 1993. p.691-719.

3. Kayhan Z. Santral bloklar. Klinik Anestezi'de genişletilmiş 3. baskı. Ankara: Logos Yayıncılık; 2005. s.552-87.

4. Morgan GE, Mikhail MS, Murray MJ, Larson CP (Çeviri: M.Tulunay, H Cuhruk). Klinik Anesteziyoloji. 3. baskı. Ankara: Güneş Kitabevi; 2004;253-81.

5. Özyalçın SN. Spinal anestezi-analjezi uygulamaları. Erdine S (Ed.). Rejyonal Anestezi'de. İstanbul: Nobel Tıp Kitabevleri; 2005. s.159-84.

6. Spielman FJ, Watson CB. Spinal anaesthesia. JAMA 1983;249:734-6.

7. A Cross National Perspective. In: ed(s). Abrams WB, Beers MH , Berkow R. The Merck Manual of Geriatrics, Whitehouse Station, N.J. Merck Research Laboratories, 1996.

8. İchley LA: Hypotension, subarachnoid block and the elderly patient. Anaesthesia 1996; 51: 1139–43.

9. Rooke GA, Freund PR, Jacobson AF: Hemodynamic response and change in organ blood volume during spinal anesthesia in elderly men with cardiac disease. Anesth Analg 1997; 85:99–105.

10. İchley LA, Stuart JC, Short TG, Gin T. Haemodynamic effects of subarachnoid block in elderly patients. Br J Anaesth 1994;73:464–70.

11. İshikawa K, Yamakage M, Omote K, Namiki A. Prophylactic IM smalldose phenylephrine blunts spinal anesthesiainduced hypotensive response during surgical repair of hip fracture in the elderly. Anesth Analg. 2002; 95: 751-756.

12. Eupre LA, Jones CA, Saunders LD, Johnston DW, Buckingham J, Majumdar SR. Best practices for elderly hip fracture patients. A systematic overview of the evidence. J Gen Intern Med. 2005; 20: 1019-1025.

13. Sheehan E, Neligan M, Murray P. Hip arthroplasty, changing trends in a national tertiary referral centre. Ir J Med Sci. 2002;171: 135.

14. Carpenter RL, Caplan RA, Brown DL, Stephenson C, Wu R. Incidence and risk factors for side effects of spinal anesthesia. Anesthesiology 1992; 76: 906–916.

15. Hoppenstein D, Zohar E, Ramaty E, Shabat S, Fredman B. The effects of general vs spinal anesthesia on frontal cerebral oxygen saturation in geriatric patients undergoing emergency surgical fixation of the neck of femur. J Clin Anesth 2005;17:431–

16. Nishikawa K, Hagiwara R, Nakamura K, Ishizeki J, Kubo K, Saito S, Goto F. The effects of the extent of spinal block on the BIS score and regional cerebral oxygen saturation in elderly patients: a prospective, randomized, and double-blinded study. J Clin Monit Comput 2007;10:109–14

17. Denault A, Deschamps A, Murkin JM. A proposed algorhythm for the intraoperative use of cerebral near-infrared spectroscopy. Semin Cardiothorac Vasc Anesth 2007;11:274-281.

18. Morgan GE, Mikhail MS, Murray MJ, Larson CP: Klinik Anesteziyoloji (LANGE), Guneş Kitabevi, Ucuncu Baskı, Ankara, 2004.S:260-269.

19. Kayhan Z.: Klinik Anestezi 3. Baskı ,Logos yayıncılık.İstanbul ,2003.**

20. Edirne S, Ozyalcın SN, Raj PP, Heavner J, Aldemir T, Yucel A: Rejyonal Anestezi. Nobel Tıp Kitabevleri, İstanbul 2005. S:159-184.

21. Lemmon WT . A method for spinal anaesthesia .Ann Surg.1940;111:144.

22. Tuohy EB.Continus spinal anaesthesia ,its usefulness and techniques involved.Anaesthesiology 1944;5:142-8.

23. Collins J.V.: Principles of Anaesthesiology.Third Edition , Lea and Febiger. Philadelphia ,Vol.2,1993.

24. Kuran O.:Sistemik Anatomi.Filiz Kitabevi.İstanbul ,1983

25. TetzlaffJ.E.:RegionalAnaesthesia&Pain Management, In "Clinical Anaesthesiology "Ed.morgan E.G.,Mikhail S.M.,Second Edition ,214-244,Appleton&Lauge ,Los Angeles ,1996.

26. Guyton C.A.:Fizyoloji .3.baskı ,Güven Kitabevi.Ankara,1993

27. Shenkman Z.,Eidelman L.A. and Cotev S.: Continuous spinal anaesthesia using a standart epidural set for extracorporeal shochware lithotripsy.Canadian Journal of Anaeshesia ; 44(10): 1042 -1046 ,1997.

28. Bernard C.M.: Epidural and Spinal Anaesthesia ,In "Anaesthesia " Ed.Barash P.G.,Third Edition,645-668,Lippincott-Raven Publishers,Philadelphia,1996.

29. Etkinson R.S.,Rushman G.B.and Davies N.J.H.: Lee"s Synopsis of Anaesthesia.Eleventh Edition.Butterwarth-Heinemann.1993

30. Kayaalp O.:Tıbbi farmakoloji ,5. baskı ,Feryal matbaacılık.Ankara ,1990.

31. Barnard M.J.,Drasner K.: Continuous spinal anaesthesia with 28 G catheter .BJA :66(3):411-412,1991.

32. Drasner K.,Sahura S.,Chan V.,Bollen A.,Ciriales R.:Persistant sacral sensory deficit induced by intrathecal local anaesthetic infusion in the rat. Anaesthesiology;80(4):847-852,1994.

33. Brian K.B.,William F.C.:Catheter spinal anaesthesia and cauda equina sydrome an lternative view. Anaesthesia &Analgesia;73(3):367-371,1991.

34. Rigler M.L.,Drasner K.,Krejcie T.C.,Yelish S.J.Scholnick F.,Defontes J.,Bohrer D.: Cauda equina sydrome after continuous spinal anaesthesia.Anaesthesia &Analgesia;72(3):275-282,1991.

35. Peyton P.,Drasner K.: Cauda equina sydrome and continuous spinal anaesthesia. Anaesthesiology;78 :214-16,1993.

36. White   PF.   Outpatient   Anaesthesia.Miller   RD,ed.   Anesthesia,   3rd   edn. NewYork:Churchill-Livingstone ,1990 :2025 -2059

37. Zauner A,Daugherty WP,Bullock MR,et al.Brainoxygenation and energy metabolism,part,1:biological function and pathophyiology.Neurosurgery.2002;51:289-302

38. Kreuzer F. Oxygen supply to tissus:the Krogh model and its asumptions.Experientia,1982;38:1415-1426

39. Micheal A.De Georgia,MD ,and Anupa Deogaonkar,:multimodal monitoring in the neurological intensive care unit 2005

40. Siesjo BK. Mechanisms of ischemic brain damage. Crit Care Med 1988;16:954-63.

41. Astrup J. Energy-requiring cell functions in the ischemic brain. Their critical supply and possible inhibition in protective therapy. J Neurosurg 1982; 56:482-97.

42. Powers WJ. Hemodynamics and metabolism in ischemic cerebrovascular disease. Neurol Clin 1992; 10:31-48.

43. Shapiro HM. Intracranial hypertension: Therapeutic and anesthetic considerations. Anesthesolgy 1975;43:445-71.)

44. Bouma GJ, Muizelaar JP. Cerebral blood flow in severe clinical head injury. New Horiz 1995;3:384-94.

45. Paulson OB, Waldemar G, Schmidt JF, Strandgaard S. Cerebral circulation under normal and pathological conditions. Am J Cardiol 1989;2:2-5.

46. Robertson CS, Cormio M. Cerebral metabolic management. New Horiz 1995;3:410-22.

47. Mc Cormick PW, Steward M, Goetting MG, Dujovny M, Lewis G, Ausman JI. Noninvasi Cerebral optical spectroscopy for monitoring cerebral oxygen delivery and hemodynamics. Crit Care Med 1991;19:89-97.

48. Messick JM Jr, Newberg LA, Nugent M, Faust RJ. Principles of neuroanaesthesia for the nonneurosurgical patient with CNS pathophysiology. Anaesth Analg 1985;64:143-74.

49. Olesen WD. Cerebral function, metabolism, and blood flow. Acta Neurol Scand 1974;57:38.

50. Aaslid R. Cerebral hemodynamics.in:Newell DW ,Aaslid R,eds .Transcranial doppler.New York,NY:1992..

51. Yonas H,Johnson D,PindzolaRR.Xenon-enhanced CT of cerebral Blood flow.Sci Am Sci med 1995;2:58-67

52. Astudillo R, van der Linden J, Ekroth R: Absent cerebral diastolic blood flow velocity after circulatory arrest but not after low flow in infants. Ann Thorac Surg. 1993; 56: 515-9.

53. Von Reutern GM, Hetzel A, Birnbaum D, Schlosser V: Transcranial Doppler ultrasonography during cardiopulmonary bypass in patients with severe carotid stenosis or occlusion. Stroke.1988; 19: 674-9.

54. Nakajima T, Kuro M, Hayashi Y, Kitaguchi K, Uchida O, Takaki O: Clinical evaluation of cerebral oxygen balance during cardiopulmonary bypass: online continuous monitoring of jugular venous oxyhemoglobin saturation. Anesth Analg. 1992; 74: 630-5.

55. Cook D, Oliver WC, Orzsulak TA, Daly RC: A prospective, randomized comparison of cerebral venous oxygen saturation during normothermic and hypothermic cardiopulmonary bypass. J Thorac Cardiovasc Surg. 1994; 107: 1020-9.

56. Ali MS, Harmer M, Vaughan R: Serum S100 protein as a marker of cerebral damage during cardiac surgery. Br J Anaesth. 2000; 85: 287-98

57. Denault A, Deschamps A, Murkin JM. A proposed algorhythm for the intraoperative use of cerebral near-infrared spectroscopy. Semin Cardiothorac Vasc Anesth 2007;11:274-281.

58. Harvey L, Edmonds HL Jr, Ganzel BL, Austin EH III. Cerebral oximetry for cardiac and vascular surgery. Semin Cardiothorac Vasc Anesth. 2004;8:147-

59. Owen-Reece H, Smith M, Elwell CE, Goldstone JC. Near infrared spectroscopy. Br J Anaesth 1999; 82: 418 – 26.

60. McCormick PW, Stewart M, Goetting MG, Dujovny M, Lewis G, Ausman JI. Noninvasive cerebral optical spectroscopy for monitoring cerebral oxygen delivery and hemodynamics. Crit Care Med 1991; 19: 89 – 97.

61. McCormick PW, Stewart M, Goetting MG, Balakrishnan G. Regional cerebrovaskular oxygen saturation measured by optical spectroscopy in human. Stroke 1991;22:596–602.

62. Olsen KS, Svendsen LB, Larsen FS. Validation of transcranial near infraredspectroscopy for evaluation of cerebral blood flow autoregulation. J Neurosurg Anesthesiol 1996;8:280 -5.

63. Madsen PL, Secher NH. Near-infrared oximetry of the brain. Prog Neurobiol 1999; 58:541 – 60.

64. Kurth CD, Thayer WS. A multiwavelength frequency-domainnear-infrared cerebral oximeter. Phys Med Biol 1999;44:727–40.

65. Williams IM, Picton AJ, Hardy SC, et al. Cerebral hypoxia detected by near infrared spectroscopy. Anaesthesia 1994;49:762–6.

66. Edmonds HL. Multi-modality neurophysiologic monitoring for cardiac surgery. Heart Surg Forum 2002; 5: 225–228.

67. Harel F, Denault A, Ngo Q, Dupis J, Khairy P. Near-infrared spectroscopy to monitor peripheral blood flow perfusion. J Clin Monit Comput 2008; 22:37-

68. Ono S, Arimitsu S, Ogawa T, Manabe H, Onoda K, Tokunaga K, et al. Continuous evaluation of regional oxygen saturation in cerebral vasospasm after subarachnoid haemorrhage using INVOS, portable near infrared spectrography. Acta Neurochir Suppl 2008;104: 215-18.

69. Harvey L, Edmonds HL Jr, Ganzel BL, Austin EH III. Cerebral oximetry for cardiac and vascular surgery. Semin Cardiothorac Vasc Anesth. 2004;8:147-
166.

70. Wahr JA, Tremper KK, Samra S, Delpy DT. Near-infrared spectroscopy: theory and applications. J Cardiothorac Vasc Anesth. 1996;10:406-18.

71. Watzman HM, Kurth CD, Montenegro LM, Rome J, Steven JM, Nicolson SC. Arterial and venous contributions to near-infrared cerebral oximetry.Anesthesiology. 2000;93:947-53.

72. Benni PB, Chen B, Dykes FD, Wagoner SF, Heard M, Tanner AJ, Young TL, Rais-Bahrami K, Rivera O, and Short BL, CAS Medical Systems, Inc., Children's National Medial Center, Washington, DC Validation of the CAS neonatal NIRS system by monitoring VV-ECMO patients: preliminary results. Advances in Experimental Medicine and Biology 2005; 566: 195-201.

73. İde K,Boushel R,Sorensen HM,Fernandes A :Department of Anaesthesia, The Copenhagen Muscle Research Centre, University of Copenhagen: 2000 170(1) 3-8

74. 1999: Ide K; Gulløv A L; Pott F; Van Lieshout J J; Koefoed B G; Petersen P; Secher N H Middle cerebral artery blood velocity during exercise in patients with atrial fibrillation. Clinical physiology (Oxford, England) 1999;19(4):284-9.

75. Collins VJ: Spinal Analgesia-Physiolgic Effects. in: Principles of Anestesiology.3rd ed. Lea&Febiger, Philadelphia, 1993, Vol:2,Sec:1498-1517.

76. Terence M: Spinal, Epidural and Caudal Anesthesia. in: Anesthesia 2nd ed, Miller RD(ed), Churchill Livingston, London, 1986,Vol:2, 1061-1106.

77. Cook DJ, Oliver WC Jr, Orszulak TA, et al. Cardiopulmonary bypass temperature, hematocrit, and cerebral oxygen delivery in humans. Ann Thorac Surg 1995; 60:1671–1677.

78. Hino A, Ueda S, Mizukawa N, et al. Effect of hemodilution on cerebral hemodynamics and oxygen metabolism. Stroke 1992; 23:423–426.

79. Sungurtekin H, Cook DJ, Orszulak TA, et al. Cerebral response to hemodilution during hypothermic cardiopulmonary bypass in adults.Anesth Analg 1999; 89:1078–1083.

80. 1998: Ide K; Pott F; Van Lieshout J J; Secher N H Middle cerebral artery blood velocity depends on cardiac output during exercise with a large muscle mass. Acta physiologica Scandinavica 1998;162(1):13-20.

81. Middle cerebral artery blood velocity during exercise in patients with atrial fibrillation Ide[1],Gulløv[2], Pott[1], J. J. Van Lieshout[3], Koefoed[2], Petersen[2], Secher[1]Article first published online: 28 JUN 2008 :150; 150-156

82. Todd MM, Wu B, Maktabi M, Hindman BJ, Warner DS: Cerebral blood flow and oxygen delivery during hypoxemia and hemodilution: role of arterial oxygen content. Am J Physiol 1994 Nov; 267(5 Pt 2):H2025-31

83. Hino A, Ueda S, Mizukawa N, et al. Effect of hemodilution on cerebral hemodynamics and oxygen metabolism. Stroke 1992; 23:423–426.

84. Marion DW, Puccio A, Wisniewski SR, et al. Effect of hyperventilation on extracellular concentrations of glutamate, lactate, pyruvate, and local cerebral blood flow in patients with severe traumatic brain injury. Crit Care Med. 2002;30:2619–2625.

85. Jens Soukup, MD, Isa Bramsiepe, MD,* Evaluation of a Bedside Monitor of Regional CBFas a Measure of CO2 Reactivity in Neurosurgical Intensive Care Patients 2008:20;249-255

86. Bengtsson M, Edström HH,Lötsröm JB,Spinal analgesia with bupivacaine,mepivacaine and tetracaine.Acta Anaesthesiol Scand 1983;27:278-283.

87.H.H Edström,PHD,C.D.Blitt,E.D.Draper Hypotansion in spinal anesthesia 1986 ;24

88. McCrae AF, Wildsmith JAW. Prevention and treatment of hypotension during central block. Br J Anaesth 1993;70: 672-680.

89. Karim Asehnoune , Eric Lorousse ,Jean mark Tadie Small dose bupivacaine –sulfentanyl prevents cardiak output after spinal anesthesia 2005 aneasthesia and analgesia :101;1512-1519

90. Kelly, J. D. *; McCoy, D. +; Rosenbaum, S. H. [P]; Brull, S. J. ++ European Journal of Anaesthesiology. 22(9):717-722, September 2005. Haemodynamic changes induced by hyperbaric bupivacaine during lateral decubitus or supine spinal anaesthesia.

91.David Hoppenstein,Edna Zohar,Erez Ramaty,Shay Shabat The Effects of Versus Spinal Anesthesia on Frontal Cerebral Oxygen Saturation in Geriatric Patients Undergoing Emergency Surgical Fization of Neck of Femur J Clin anest 17;431-438,2205

92. Vincent Minville,Karim Asehnoune,Sabrina Salau,Bernard Tissot The Effects of Spinal Anesthesia on Cerebral Blood Flow in Very Elderly   Anesth and Analgesia 2009 ;108-129:1291-4

93. Koichi Nishikawa,Ryuji Hagiwara,Kohji Nakamura,Junko İshizeki Journal of Clinical Monitoring and Computing 2007 21:109-114

94.Gustafson Y,Berggren D,Brannströn G,Norberg A. Acute confusional states in elderly patients treated for femoral neck fracture .J Am Geriatr Soc 1988 ;36:525-30

95. Neilson WR, Gelb AW, Casey JE, Penny FJ. long term cognitive and social sequelae of general versus regional anesthesia during arthroplasty in the elderly. Anesthesiology;1990:73; 103-109

96. Yao FS, Tseng CC, Ho CY, Levin SK, Illner P. Cerebral oxygen desaturation is associated with early postoperative neuropsychological dysfunction in patients undergoing cardiac surgery. J Cardiothorac Vasc Anesth 2004;18:552-8.

97. Folstein MF, Folstein SE, McHugh PR. "Mini-mental state".A practical method for grading the cognitive state of patientsfor the clinician. J Psychiatr Res 1975;12:189-98.

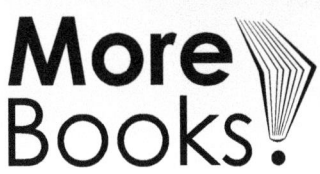
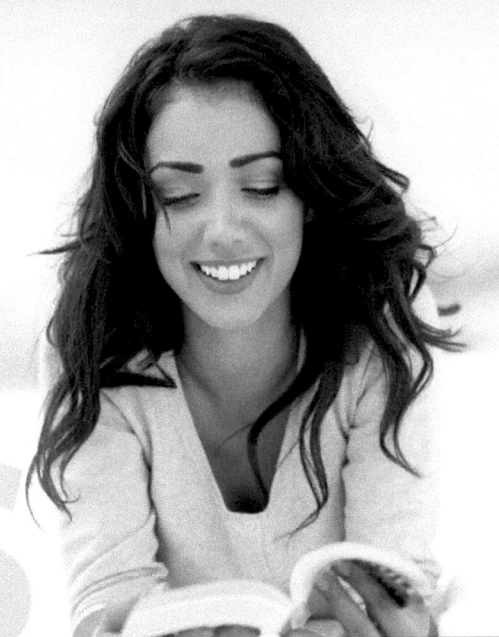

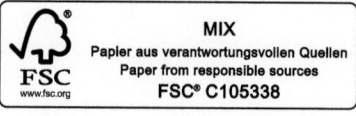